Praise for *Matters of the Mouth*

"This book is an indispensable tool in the pursuit of health. Just read it. You won't be sorry."

—Ty Bollinger, author and founder of *The Truth About Cancer* and *The Truth About Vaccines*

"*Matters of the Mouth* leaves no stone unturned when it comes to revealing the secrets to living a healthy lifestyle for optimal health. This book has all of the answers you need; everyone should read it."

—Kristin Cavallari, TV personality and entrepreneur

"*Matters of the Mouth* finally connects all the dots of holistic health. If you are looking for a comprehensive book that addresses the multitude of health issues we all face, especially the conditions of the mouth which are commonly ignored, this book is for you. Dr. Thom doesn't just tell you all the problems like many other health books out there, he gives you solutions to start changing your health that you can start applying immediately. This book is a must-have for understanding how optimal health is achieved and maintained so that we can live our lives to the fullest! A must-buy!"

—Courtland Nall, RDH, IBDM, holistic hygienist

"Dr. Thom understands that the mouth is the doorway to our health, and that inflammation and nutrition aren't just important for the body, but also for our dental health. He is one of the cutting-edge leaders in the natural dentist movement. That is why I have endorsed him as one of the top 50 Functional & Integrative Medical Doctors in America."

—Dr. Josh Axe, DNM, DC, CNS, founder of Ancient Nutrition

"*Matters of the Mouth* will be your guide to transform the health of your teeth and gums, which can lead to a lifetime of 'whole-body' wellness."

—Jordan Rubin, founder of Garden of Life and Ancient Nutrition and *New York Times* bestselling author of *The Maker's Diet*

"*Matters of the Mouth* is a comprehensive health how-to for our times. Dr. Lokensgard lifts the veil to help the reader realize the delicate intricacies and interconnections of the mouth as a circuit breaker for the entire body and thus the awesome, personal responsibility we assume with our choices. *Matters of the Mouth* encapsulates the inescapable reality that what we allow into our mouth—both dental work or nutrition—is a two-edged sword, helping or harming us with every bite."

—Scott Laird, ND, founder of LairdWellness.com and host of *The Health Awakening* podcast

"Dr. Thom's unique approach to wellness, healing, rejuvenation, and antiaging is a game changer. *Matters of the Mouth* is not to be missed. . . . It's to be read and reread and highlighted and underlined with notes taken in the margins."

—Leigh-Allyn Baker, actress and health advocate

"Dr. Lokensgard's mastery of the full gamut of issues that can influence and restore human health is beautifully presented in *Matters of the Mouth*. The reader will learn ways to decrease their chances of getting sick and ways to screen health practitioners to ensure they are using the powerful healing principles of biological medicine and dentistry, natural methods that work to restore true lasting health. *Matters of the Mouth* is an informative read for both the layperson and healthcare professionals."

—David A. Jernigan, BSc Nutrition, DNM, DC, Biologix Center for Optimum Health

"*Matters of the Mouth* is an encyclopedia of knowledge that is a must-have for every home. Dr. Thom's understanding of the relationship of oral health to overall health is shared here with practical advice and is hard to put down. This book should be read and reread."

—Joe Doctora, DDS, MD, associate professor, Deptartment of Oral and Maxillofacial Surgery, School of Dentistry, Meharry Medical College; co-founder of Pearl Oral Health

MATTERS OF THE MOUTH

A Holistic Guide to Achieving Optimal Oral and Overall Health

Thomas Lokensgard, DDS, NMD, ABAAHP
with Greg Webster

Foreword by Del Bigtree
Foreword by Ty Bollinger

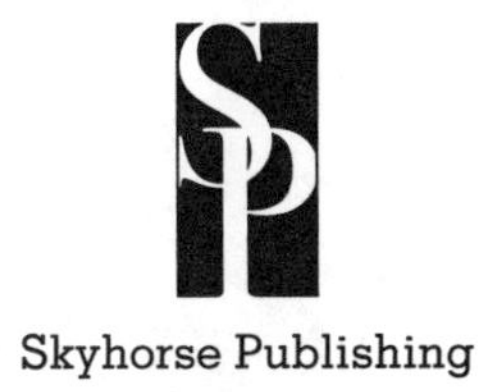

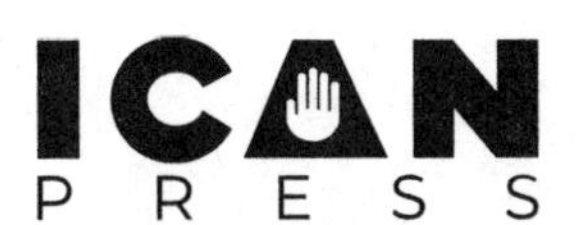

Skyhorse Publishing books may be purchased in bulk at special discounts for sales promotion, corporate gifts, fund-raising, or educational purposes. Special editions can also be created to specifications. For details, contact the Special Sales Department, Skyhorse Publishing, 307 West 36th Street, 11th Floor, New York, NY 10018 or info@skyhorsepublishing.com.

Visit our website at www.skyhorsepublishing.com.

Please follow our publisher Tony Lyons on Instagram @tonylyonsisuncertain.

10 9 8 7 6 5 4 3 2 1

Library of Congress Cataloging-in-Publication Data is available on file.

Cover design by David Ter-Avanesyan
Cover photograph by Getty Images

Print ISBN: 978-1-64821-092-1
Ebook ISBN: 978-1-64821-093-8

Printed in the United States of America

Disclaimer

The content of this book is provided for information purposes only. The author does not assume any liability to any person for the information or advice (or the use of such information or advice) which is provided in this book or incorporated into it by reference. The information is provided on the basis that all persons will undertake responsibility for assessing the relevance and accuracy of its content. It is not meant to be used, nor should it be used, to diagnose or treat any medical condition. For diagnosis or treatment of any medical problem, consult your own physician. The author is not responsible for any specific health or allergy needs that may require medical supervision and is not liable for any damages or negative consequences from any treatment, action, application, or preparation to any person reading or following the information in this manual.

This book is not intended as a substitute for the medical advice of physicians, dentists, naturopaths, chiropractors, or qualified healthcare practitioners. The reader should regularly consult with a dentist, physician, or licensed and qualified practitioner, in matters relating to his or her health and particularly with respect to any symptoms that may require diagnosis or medical attention.

The information provided in this book is designed to provide helpful information on the subjects discussed.

References are provided for informational purposes only and do not constitute endorsement of any websites or other sources.

You are advised to work with a qualified healthcare practitioner licensed in your State and in their field of endeavor.

Contents

Foreword by Del Bigtree *xiii*

Foreword by Ty Bollinger *xv*

Introduction **xvii**

Diving into My Career

Something's Missing

Do What You Love!

Patience and Patients Are Great Teachers

Another Love

Your Number One Asset

What's Food Got to Do with It?

PART ONE: YOUR MOUTH AS AN INDICATOR OF YOUR HEALTH

Chapter 1—How Are Functional Dentistry and Integrative Medicine Related? **3**

What Is Biological or Functional Dentistry?

The Roots of Health

Biological Systems vs. Biological Stressors

The Biological Terrain

Cellular Healing Protocol

The Secret of Cellular Metabolic Medicine

Modern Medical and Dental Myopic Myths

Chapter 2—Total Health Begins in Your Mouth **19**

Mouthing Off

The Heart-Periodontal Link

Bodily Enemy #1 Dental Decay

The Dentinal Fluid Transport System (DFTS)

Bodily Enemy #2 Gingivitis and #3 Periodontal Disease

The Alzheimer's Disease Connection

Natural Prevention and Healing of Gingivitis and Periodontal Disease

What Causes Bad Breath?

Chapter 3—Making Your Mouth Healthy Again 35
The Oral Pauses of Life Medical Model
Saliva and Its Function
The Lymph Connection
The Problem with Osteo-Cavitations
The Urinary Filtrate
The Truth About Root Canals
Biofilm, Bacteria, Nutritional Deficiencies, and Dental Decay

Chapter 4—What Is Antiaging Medicine and Dentistry? 49
The Importance of Free Radical Oxidation
The Optimal Health Continuum
Age Rejuvenation: A Legacy of Good Health
Prevention and Aging
Functional Jaw Orthopedic Orthodontics
What Is Craniofacial Orthopedics?
Eight Keys to Facial Beauty and TMJ Health
Orthodontics: Three-Phase Treatment
Craniosacral Therapy
How Do We Move Teeth Orthodontically?

PART TWO: PRINCIPLES OF ANTI-AGING AND FUNCTIONAL MEDICINE

Chapter 5—Optimum Oral Health for Life 65
Ozone: An (Oxygen) Blast from the Past
Zeolites: What Are They, and How Do They Function?
The Amazing Benefits of Oil Pulling
How to Clean Your Teeth Naturally
A Special Word about Your Baby's Teeth
What's Good for You? Serum Compatibility Testing

Chapter 6—A Little TLC for the TMJ 75
What is TMJ Disorder?
Self-Care for TMJD
Bruxism, Grinding, Malocclusion, and Mineral Deficiency

Chapter 7—The War on Inflammation 79
Breaking the Silence
Health Education: The Prescription for Disease Prevention
The Fat Factor
Anti-Inflammatory Eating
The Glycemic Index (GI) and Glycemic Load (GL)
Biblical Nutrition

Chapter 8—The Good, the Bad, and the Beneficial 93
The Benefits of Raw Milk
Iodine and Its Importance
The Acidic-Alkaline Shift
The Assault on Salt

Chapter 9—It's a Toxic World 105
Toxins All Around
The Toxic Results
The Politics of the Food Industry and the GMO Dilemma
Refined Sugar, the Modern-Day Toxin
The Safe Sugars List
The Benefits of Clean Water

Chapter 10—OSA and Insomnia—Why Can't I Sleep? 117
Obstructive Sleep Apnea (OSA)
Arrested Rest
Treat Yourself to a Good Night's Sleep

PART THREE: SOLUTIONS TO COMMON HEALTH PROBLEMS

Chapter 11—The Fattening of America 125
The Lowdown on Low-Fat
The Battle with Food Manufacturers
The Low-Fat Diet Myth

Chapter 12—Controlling Chronic Constipation 133
Attack the Cause, Solve the Problem
Colon Nourishment

Chapter 13—The Candida Conundrum 137
CRC: The Candida-Related Complex
The Great Mimicker
Symptoms of Candidiasis
And the Solution Is?
Natural Yeast Fighters
Repair after the Battle's Won

Chapter 14—Heavy Metal and Whole-Body Detoxification 147
Mercury and Other Toxic Conspirators
The Oral Rejuvenation, Heavy Metal Detoxification Plan
The Importance of Safe Mercury Amalgam Removal
The Special Role of Glutathione in Detoxification
The Importance of Chelation Therapy
How Your Body Detoxifies

Do You Need to Detox?
Special Case #1: Detoxing for Weight Control
Special Case #2: Detoxing for Autism Healing

PART FOUR: KEY SOLUTIONS FOR WHOLE-BODY HEALTH AND ANTIAGING MEDICINE

Chapter 15—The Whole-Health Lifestyle **163**
Become Anti-Antibiotics and Pro-Probiotics
Optimize Your Whole-Body Systems
Remineralize Your Life, Teeth, and Skeletal Matrix
The Special Case of Breastfeeding
Dental Meridians

Chapter 16—A Final Look at Your Teeth **171**
The Importance of Fixing Crooked Teeth the Right Way
The Big Takeaways

Chapter 17—What About Dentistry and Cancer? **175**
Cancer Prevention
Folic Acid and Cancer
Boron and Cancer
Cancer Supplementation
Natural Cancer Therapies

Appendix 1—Anti-Inflammatory Foods **185**
Appendix 2—Alkaline Foods **189**
Appendix 3—Mercury Toxicity Sensitivity Questionnaire **191**
Appendix 4—TMJ Self-Assessment Questionnaire **193**
Appendix 5—CR or Caloric Reduction **195**
Appendix 6—Meridian Tooth Chart **197**
Appendix 7—Probiotic and Prebiotic Instructions **199**
Appendix 8—Dirty Dozen and the Clean 15 **201**
Appendix 9—A Final Word **203**
Appendix 10—The Life Rejuvenation Programs **205**

Acknowledgments *207*

Index *209*

Foreword

by Del Bigtree

Growing up, my parents were always the most radical health nuts in town. We didn't have any of the "fun foods" that my friends had like Doritos, Fruit Loops, or Coca Cola . . . ever. Do you know what it's like to try and trade a bowl of tabbouleh for a bologna on Wonder Bread sandwich in elementary school? I do. It's impossible! I remember one day when I threatened my mother that it could be considered child abuse to deny me the experience of a lollipop. She agreed and returned moments later with a prune on a toothpick.

Shockingly, despite the absolute dearth of refined sugar in my adolescence, I still got cavities and went to the dentist like every other kid. I remember other parents warning mine that denying me access to sugar would only create a longing that could lead to addiction in adulthood. But as an adult, I can confidently say that that never happened. I have always craved less sugar than others around me, and, by and large, have been attracted to a healthier diet than most of my friends.

I honestly thought that I had been given the tools to live forever. But when I turned forty, I started having issues with inflammation in my joints and my stomach, and I felt fatigued more than seemed reasonable. Many would say, "You're just getting old." But I knew there had to be a better explanation.

In 2016, I met Thomas Lokensgard and his wife, Jan, at a gathering at the Herban Market in Franklin, Tennessee, for my film *Vaxxed*. The following year, we met again in Nashville at an event for *The Truth About Cancer*, hosted by our mutual friends Ty and Charlene Bollinger.

Thom is one of those guys you find yourself telling your life story to before you've even finished shaking hands. I couldn't believe how knowledgeable he was about the human body. I remember asking, "What is it you do again?" He replied, "I'm a dentist." Thom began to explain that many of the health issues I was having could not be changed by diet or by exercise because the poison I was trying to detoxify was lodged in my teeth.

As it turns out, some of the decisions that my parents had made with my dentist as a child were killing me as an adult. Because I had a few baby teeth that never fell out, the mercury they had been filled with was leaching into my body.

I was also surprised to discover that the root canals I'd had as a young adult were priming me for a heart attack.

Over the next year, I made many trips to Thom's office in Nashville, where we carefully removed all the toxins from my mouth. With each trip, I became more and more enamored with his encyclopedic knowledge of all of the systems of the body and the simple household remedies that could bring everything back into alignment.

I was sad when Thom decided to retire from dentistry, not because I'd lost the best dentist I'd ever had, but because I'd lost one of the best healers. I realize now that his retirement just gave him the time to write this incredible book so the world could share in his wisdom.

Matters of the Mouth is more than a book about oral health; it is a manual for optimal health. I would never have been healthy enough to fly around the world and do the work that I am so passionate about without Thom. Let me be the first to introduce you to one of my secret weapons.

Foreword

by Ty Bollinger

Is fluoride good for your teeth?
Are root canals safe?
Is there mercury in most dental fillings?

The answer to these questions might surprise you. The truth is that most of what you've been taught about oral health and medicine isn't factually true. It's based on folklores that have their roots in corporate greed with the goal of creating lifelong "customers" for drug companies and the "healthcare" industry (which should more appropriately be called the "sickness perpetuation" industry).

The lies surrounding the dental industry are pervasive, persistent, and widely accepted. As a general rule, it's rare that you find a dentist who is more educated than most doctors about matters of true health and healing. Dr. Thomas Lokensgard is the exception to the rule. And in this groundbreaking book—*Matters of the Mouth*—he shares much of that knowledge with the reader. Dr. Thom has been our family dentist for almost eight years, and it's because of his thorough knowledge of oral health that I have my periodontal disease under control.

If you want to be vibrantly healthy, you must consider the importance of oral health. In this book, you'll learn the truth about many vital topics, including:

- The importance of functional dentistry and integrative medicine
- How to slow down the aging process through free radical oxidation
- Chronic inflammation and degenerative disease
- The importance of beneficial bacteria
- How to avoid and eliminate toxins in our food, water, and environment
- The truth about root canals and TMJ
- The connection between dentistry and cancer
- How to optimize your oral health

And so much more!

It's time for us to overcome the lies and awaken to the higher truth that we have all been lied to about almost everything related to health, especially oral health. There is a better way to approach oral well-being and disease prevention, and it doesn't involve making Big Pharma companies rich while the people suffer. Instead, it's based on potent prevention strategies, healing exposure to natural molecules (like ozone), minimizing exposure to toxins and other causes of inflammation, and many other practical practices outlined in *Matters of the Mouth.*

Once you jettison the systematic poisons and toxins, while simultaneously increasing your body's natural defenses, immune system, and detoxification pathways, you will experience a significant increase in your oral health, overall consciousness, and quality of life.

Introduction

I have always been especially fascinated by the sciences. In grade school, I entered the science fair and came away with a blue ribbon for my project, "The Human Body." From early on, there were three things I always wondered about:

1. What did it look like at the bottom of a lake?
2. What did the inside of the human body look like?
3. How did the body work?

My passion for science led me into a career in dentistry and medicine, and as I grew older, I had the opportunity to satisfy my first two curiosities. The third, though, involves the amazing intricacy of how our physical bodies operate, and as much as I've learned about its wonders since I was a kid, I will likely spend the rest of my life discovering new and fascinating aspects of how we're put together. But even my discoveries in answering the first two questions are a significant part of my journey in medicine and dentistry.

Diving into My Career

I was trained and certified in rescue and advanced scuba diving in the mid-1990s and have since seen the bottom of quite a few lakes, including Lake Superior where I very nearly lost my life seventy feet below the surface, while exploring the wreck of the *Madeira*. The *Madeira* sank off the coast of Two Harbors, Minnesota, in a severe late-autumn storm in 1905 and has been the subject of a number of explorations since the 1950s. Mike, a Navy diving buddy of mine, and I set out to explore the sunken pilot house one day in 1996, right after I received my advanced scuba-diving certificate as I had just finished the PADI advanced scuba certification a month prior.

It was Memorial Day, and we were diving in thirty-four-degree Lake Superior waters. I had just purchased a new regulator which, I had been told, needed an environmental kit to prevent freeze-up in cold water. The salesman at the dive shop had said, no problem, you can just put it on when you come back. At 70 feet, I had fully exhaled on my way to 120 feet, where the wheelhouse was resting. I realized quickly that I had no air and that my backup regulator was also frozen up. I grabbed Mike's foot, just in time, and he gave me his spare air, thus saving my life. I had wanted to rocket quickly to the surface, but he kept a slow pace.

Rising too fast while holding your breath can cause your lungs to explode via lung over-pressurization. This is the most common cause of death during diving expeditions.

Upon our return to the dive shop, the sales rep called US Divers and they said the step-down port had most likely frozen, developed ice crystals, and blocked the air intake port because I should have had an environmental kit in place. Afterward, I told Mike that I'd continue diving but we needed to become rescue certified. My near-death experience in the waters of Lake Superior alerted me to the value of life and what I should do to make each day count.

In 1974, I had received a bachelor's degree from Concordia College in Moorhead, Minnesota. True to my long-standing passion, I majored in biology with special emphasis in biochemistry and physiology. Even while attending college, I did what I could to follow my passion and found many answers to my second question working as an autopsy assistant for a pathology group at Fairview-Southdale Hospital in Edina, Minnesota, where I lived during two of my college years.

Although I was accepted into the endocrinology program at Colorado State College, I opted instead to enter dentistry school at the University of Minnesota and graduated in December 1979 with a DDS degree. A month later, I started my dental career in Park Rapids, Minnesota, with an emphasis in cosmetic restorative dentistry and orthopedic orthodontics. In the years that followed, my interest and knowledge in orthodontic and craniofacial procedures deepened as I took hundreds of additional hours in continuing education credits in those disciplines.

Something's Missing

In the early 1990s, I began to sense that something was missing in traditional medicine and dentistry. I had begun to believe there was a connection between nutrition and wellness, and I questioned the prescribing of pharmaceuticals for what seemed like any and every symptom that presented itself in the doctor's office.

As I continued my studies and observed what was happening with my own patients, it became increasingly clear there was an undeniable connection between nutrition and optimal health. Several key areas of biomarkers seemed especially pertinent, and I began to explore nutritional, probiotic, glyconutrient, enzyme, and endocrine therapies. I also joined the American Nutraceutical Association (ANA) in 2001. Through my connections there, I discovered a body of new scientific information that completely supported my new way of thinking about helping patients achieve optimal health.

One study in particular—a Harvard Medical School study*—helped connect the last few dots for me. The Harvard research revealed a clear link between

* Harvard Medical School, "Treating gum disease may lessen the burden of heart disease, diabetes, other conditions." Heart Health, 2014. http://www.health.harvard.edu/blog/treating-gum-disease-may-lessen-burden-heart-disease-diabetes-conditions-201407237293.

a widespread condition called "silent inflammation" and periodontitis disease (inflammation of tissue around the teeth) and heart disease—two very important American health issues.

In 2003, I completed training in Botox® and dermal fillers, entered the field of cosmetic facial aesthetics, and started OralMed Aesthetics in Minneapolis. The new direction in my thinking about the modern medical paradigm so energized me that I just couldn't get enough of it, so in 2004, I entered the Naturopathic Medical Doctoral Program at Clayton College of Natural Health in Birmingham, Alabama. The course of study, open only to practitioners with doctoral degrees, gave me the foundation for a nutritionally based dentistry practice. This was revolutionary. After all, how many dentists have you heard of who include nutrition as part of their dental health programs? Yet, I had discovered that whole-body nutrition is fundamental to good dental—as well as every other aspect of—health.

By 2009, my thirty years of clinical experience and membership in the American Academy of AntiAging Medicine (A4M) enabled me to become board-certified in AntiAging Medicine as a Diplomate (that's where the "ABAAHP" after my name comes from). More recently, I've completed a fellowship program offered by the A4M and continue my quest to answer the third question every day: How does the body work?

Do What You Love!

At the University of Northern Colorado, my college roommate, Bob, was an opera singer. I, on the other hand, was an acoustic guitar player and although I loved the music of Crosby, Stills, Nash, and Young, Bob hated it and let me know how he felt almost daily. While he sang on the university stage, I played the acoustic pop scene—coffeehouses, pubs, homespun restaurants. Bob loved opera, and I didn't. And I still don't. My family and I watched *The Voice* and still enjoy acoustic pop music together.

The difference between Bob and me, though, demonstrates a serious life principle that we all need to embrace. Each of us is designed with a unique combination of gifts, desires, and abilities that make up our calling in life. The beauty of it is that to find and follow that calling allows us to do the very thing we most want to do and were designed to do.

This principle came into sharp focus for me thanks to my undergraduate biology professor at the University of Northern Colorado. When I discovered his personal background, his presence at the school became a mystery to me. He was a surgeon who had been trained at Baylor University but was teaching a freshman biology class. Since he was also my academic advisor, I developed a close enough personal relationship that I eventually mustered the nerve to ask him why he traded surgery for teaching undergraduate biology students. His answer resonated with me then and has been a guiding principle for me ever since: "If you're not happy with what you're doing," he said, "then you should do what you love—and I love to teach."

So, I love music, sports, scuba diving, teaching, and science. Fortunately for me, I've been captivated by science since before I even knew what the scientific method was, so pursuing the study of science far beyond freshman biology has been a natural path for me. When I was accepted into the University of Minnesota dentistry program, my foray into the world of Western science deepened dramatically, but often because of troubling observations as much as from good teaching. For instance, a well-respected biochemist once told our biochemistry class that, "In America, we could never have macro- or micronutrient deficiencies because we have vitamin-enriched bread, like Wonder Bread."

At the time I assumed that since I was paying a lot of money for an elite professional education, whatever I was being taught must be true, right? But I quickly discovered how wrong that assumption was.

While attending dentistry school, I discussed some of my growing suspicions with Dr. James O. Beck, chairman of the oral radiology program. A distinguished oral pathologist and oral radiologist, he listened intently to what I had to say about the imperfections in the dentistry curriculum. Then he looked at me and said, "Thomas, I know there are a few of you who are frustrated, but I want you to remember one thing: It doesn't matter what they do to you; what matters is how you respond." He was right, and it opened my thinking to another critical mindset that has guided my search for the truth in medical research and treatment.

In today's world, you have two choices that can get you into trouble:

1. You can ignore the truth, or
2. You can believe a lie.

Either one will bring you to the wrong result or conclusion!

Here are three examples:

1. Cable and network news are owned by Big Pharma and Big Agribusiness. Don't believe me? Watch the advertising. Morning, noon, and night, 24/7.
2. Mainstream, symptom-based medicine is alternative because it is alternative to God's physiology and His Grand Design. Symptom-based medicine is alternative, because it too, is alternative to normal human physiology.
3. Natural health is not alternative, it's physiologic, because it enhances normal human physiology and enhances your health by balancing your organ systems biochemically and bioenergetically.

Remember, you cannot pharmacologically intoxicate someone into health.

My friend and first accountant, Edric Clarke, used to hammer into my head that, "Winners get knocked down nine times, but they get up ten, while losers get knocked down nine times only to get up eight." An avid Scouter, Edric asked me to serve as Scoutmaster in a local troop and eventually invited me into the BSA Eagle Board of Review. He, too, added a meaningful component to my thinking with his practical advice: "Do not die trying to bring a great idea to perfection." Sometimes, it is fine to take what you do know and act on it rather than waiting for the indefinite—and unrealistic—goal of achieving perfection before "trying anything." As a result, I've taken a learn-as-you-go approach to my work.

Patience and Patients Are Great Teachers

When I began practicing dentistry in 1980, I realized early on that I could learn something from all of my patients. I wondered, for instance, why some patients had terrible habits and yet manifested no adverse health implications, while others with great habits experienced all kinds of health complications. I became determined to better understand the connection between health, nutrition, and disease, so I joined the American Nutraceutical Association (ANA) and the American Academy of Anti-Aging Medicine (A4M) and began working on my Naturopathic Medical Doctorate (NMD) degree.

Through these associations, I discovered a group of like-minded doctors who saw the nutritional connection I was looking for and had a hunch that it truly existed. Among other things, I was not alone in beginning to question the wisdom of placing mercury fillings in people's teeth—especially close to the blood-brain barrier. I hadn't yet heard of biological dentistry, but was on my way. I had begun to realize that approximately half of what I'd been taught in the dentistry program was wrong, I just needed to figure out which half.

While practicing in Minnesota, I had one particular patient who had been on her own search for a better means to good health. Upon introducing herself, she handed me a printout and said, "Here is a list of the forty-nine doctors I've visited, and you are number fifty." She was dead serious and wanted real answers. So, I referred her to a bioenergetic chiropractic specialist, whom I had met recently. I found out later that he diagnosed a cavitation (a hole in the bone) in the third molar position, which had bothered her for years, and, despite being an experienced dentist by then, it was the first time I had heard of such a thing. I realized immediately that I needed to bring my diagnostic skills up to speed, and my journey into biological dentistry and medicine accelerated dramatically.

Perhaps the greatest contributor of all to this new endeavor has been my wife, Jan. While everyone else was eating sugar and white bread, drinking Tang and decaffeinated coffee, Jan was into organic whole wheat, honey, smoothies, garden vegetables, and raw milk. She was so far ahead of her time that once during a short stay in the hospital, she requested real oatmeal, whole wheat bread, bananas, orange juice, and yogurt, instead of pudding, skim milk, soda pop, sugar cereal, and pastries. The hospital dietician sent a staff member to the grocery store to purchase it for her because the hospital kitchen didn't stock such nutritious fare.

Another Love

"In 1999, I recorded a contemporary Christian, pop, acoustic vocal record at a studio in Los Angeles, put a band together, and toured around the Upper Midwest. The band was called the Thomas Jordan Band, after myself and son Jordan, who was the bass player. We received modest attention from radio play in thirty-eight states and I really enjoyed our (admittedly short) run. The album and title song is called *Day by Day* and is available on Spotify by Thomas Jordan.

During this time, I sold my first dental practice in Park Rapids, Minnesota, and moved my family to Minneapolis. In 2008, Jan and I landed in Franklin, Tennessee, where my holistic dental career really took off. We both loved it there—and so did our family. Today, our kids and their families live in various states."

My reason for sharing this part of my story with you is twofold. First, I want you to know where I've come from professionally and personally in hopes you'll be encouraged by the necessity of taking the time and effort to pursue something meaningful. And secondly, I hope you will reflect on your own progress. Here, in brief, are my suggestions to help you evaluate yourself:

1. Where are you in your journey? We are all at different places in life, facing various struggles. That's essential to a quality journey, and you shouldn't let it stop you.
2. Follow your gut, seek the truth, pursue your passions, don't reinvent the wheel, follow the gurus, do what you love, protect your family, and most important, follow the Lord's guidance for your life.
3. And as I like to say, "It's what you learn after you know it all that really counts." Keep moving and keep learning—and forgive always!

Your Number One Asset

With so much confusion over what some refer to as healthcare delivery, the current medical model most definitely needs major revision. It is crucial that you take control of your own healthcare since, contrary to popular "spin," government has proven time and again that it cannot help you out in a crisis.

The great Greek scientist and physician Hippocrates knew two thousand years ago the fundamental key to good medicine when he taught: "Let your food be your medicine and your medicine be your food." Yet it is an idea that has been lost through the ages—especially in the "medicalization" or "sophistication" of our own time. Disconnecting good health from nutrition has also disconnected individuals from the need to take responsibility for their own health.

Medicine—and the perception of the health that it offers—has become the sole responsibility of professionals and the associated over-the-top expensive, ineffective, bureaucratic machinery paid for by a distant third-party payer. The fallout from this approach includes the dysfunctional reality that no one really knows what healthcare is actually costing our society, but suffice it to say it's way too much.

To see how far down the wrong path we have been led, check out my *32 Ways to Reverse the Aging Process.* If you're like most people, you'll be amazed at how few of these ways have been followed or recommended in the current medical paradigm. It's not surprising, though. Even the most well-intentioned practitioners have a hard time keeping up. According to the A4M, medical knowledge doubles every three and a half years, so it doesn't take much time to become out-of-date. And guess who suffers for that? Anyone who simply follows the "party line"—maybe even you. The problem is that your health is your most important personal asset, and no one should have more of a vested interest in protecting it than you!

What's Food Got to Do with It?

Food and nutrition is information for your cytoplasmic genetic switches, also known as genetic signaling molecules. In other words, food tells your hormones and genes which proteins to assemble.

When I began to connect food to good medicine, I was still living in Minnesota but had just made a trip to Nashville after joining the ANA and discovered a group of MDs, DDSs, and DCs who were plugged into a fascinating nutritional-medical model. I immediately bought in, and it changed my life and work.

My own recognition of the truth of Hippocrates's words came in an aha moment at a nutritional seminar, in which one of the speakers made this eye-opening statement: "There is a battle being waged, but it's not against your doctor, the medical establishment, nor your insurance company. The battle is being waged in the grocery store." It hit me that the piece lacking in the medical puzzle was nutritionally based, yet medically missing, and also missing from the current realm of healthcare.

This was well before I'd ever heard of genetically modified (GMO) foods or really understood much about nutrition. I think it's worth reiterating that these days, we are bombarded with medical *mis*information brought to you by way of deceptive TV advertising and pseudo-agribusiness. Numerous cable and network TV ads promote GMO and bioengineered foods and Big Pharma as healthy and "biologic." Often sponsored by organizations with a vested interest in the products under study, the research is disingenuous, at best, and at times intentionally falsified.

This, in my opinion, is the very essence of Fake News. There is nothing that is "biologic" about Humira or Jardiance or Toujeo. Where do they come up with these cute names anyway? These at best are "alternative drugs" because they are *alternative* to normal human cellular physiology and God's amazing genetic blueprint.

I've learned to look at biological systems because that is how the Creator designed us. Your mouth, for example, as the beginning of your gastrointestinal tract, is a system.

The good news is that today, there are many more forward-thinking and practicing doctors who have the same passion for natural health as I do. I'm even putting together a much larger program—far beyond the scope of this book—to help and encourage them in their practices as well as individuals like you who are serious about your health. In a nutshell, these are the key points for managing your own health. You must:[*]

- Discover that you have to take control of your own health.
- Stay committed to a lifestyle of personal responsibility (part of taking control).
- Learn optimal oral health and oral disease prevention.
- Understand whole-body systems and their intricate connections to oral and general health.
- Discover the basic testing panels that you need to optimize your overall health.
- Learn how important it is to control silent inflammation and recognize that it is the centerpiece to your well-being.[†]
- Keep up-to-date symptom checklists for you to present to your doctor with whom you should work (they are in my program).
- Proceed at your own pace, time, and cost. Study, study, study.

The distinctive aspect of the medical approach that I now advocate is to think of health issues in terms of whole-body systems. These systems must also be in balance. This is called homeostasis and is essential for our well-being. What this is not, is alternative, as it is a God-designed physiological and biological system in every sense of the word. Remember: we are biochemical as well as bioelectrical in our design and makeup.

The approach could also be called by any number of other names:

- A sickness or aging-reversal system.
- An aging-prevention program.
- A cellular-metabolic medical model focusing on cellular regeneration.

---

* You can access this information at http://www.DrLokensgard.com.

† Benedict C. Albensi, *What Is Nuclear Factor Kappa B (NF-κB) Doing in and to the Mitochondrion?*, http://www.frontiersin.org/articles/10.3389/fcell.2019.00154/full.

- A lifelong lifestyle nutritional program.
- Integrative, physiological, functional, complementary, biological, or bioenergetic.

As part of this new approach, understanding the differing values in acute care versus chronic degenerative disease (CDD) is essential. What do I mean by this? For starters, CDD care is lifestyle-oriented. Some call it antiaging medicine. I call it biological or physiological medicine. Acute care, on the other hand, happens in a crisis or an emergency situation and is what the American medical system does better than any other country in the world. For example, modern medical professionals do an astounding job of putting people back together surgically after automobile wrecks and many other traumatic accidents. Much of what is accomplished is nearly miraculous. We fail miserably, however, in understanding how to treat lifestyle disease (CDD) and that is a very, very, very big problem with the generally accepted approach to symptom-based, prescription-pad, Band-Aid medicine.

In 2018 I partnered with Dr. Joe Doctora in creating our new line of Pearl Oral Health™ care products. Together, Dr. Doctora and I have degrees in medicine, biological dentistry, oral surgery, and naturopathy, including special training in antiaging medicine. Our superior products are nontoxic, safe, effective, clinically beneficial, and essential for good health.

Our Pearl Oral Health (POH) products include Pearl Nature's Toothpaste®, which is my personal formulation, and OxyMist®, and Pearl Silica Drops® (formally known as Silidyn Rejuvenate). We are also in the process of developing a new oral probiotic that will further enhance the oral microbiome.

Visit our website for more information.*

* http://www.PearlOralHealth.com.

PART ONE

Your Mouth as an Indicator of Your Health

CHAPTER 1

How Are Functional Dentistry and Integrative Medicine Related?

This is a very different and more comprehensive approach to your health and it requires a lot more effort and scrutiny on your part. You must begin this journey, like I did mine, by analyzing what you have been taught through deceitful and misguided TV commercials and a pharmaceutical industry that wants you to believe in the "magic bullet" theory.

If you have trouble buying into what I am saying, then put down the GMO groceries that you just purchased and start doing your own homework. Start with your habits and focus.

A Colorado pastor stated something that I found extremely interesting. Scripturally, he said, "Man was created as a habitual being, not a disciplined being."

People do not decide their future, they decide their focus. The focus then creates the habit, and your habits decide your future. This has enormous implications with regard to changing your lifestyle habits and can be directly applied to taking control of your own health.

The assumption here is that in order to accomplish your goals, it is going to take a lot of hard work to break your habitual patterns and replace them with the discipline you need. This is extremely powerful stuff.

Integrative medicine and functional dentistry are the fields of healthcare that focus on:

- Augmenting DNA repair through nutrition
- Biochemical individuality
- Cellular metabolic balance
- Dietary endocrinology
- Environmental toxic content. Detoxifying the body.
- Genetic predisposition and expression
- Genetic SNPs testing
- Individualized nutraceutical and nutritional analysis

- Individual nutritional prescriptions
- Lifestyle patterns and how to change them for better health
- Metabolic and nutritional profiles
- Natural hormonal and neurotransmitter optimization
- Nutritional balance
- Prevention of disease at the cellular metabolic level
- Silent inflammation control
- Stress management and parasympathetic and sympathetic nervous system control

Better to wear out than to rust out.
—Jack LaLanne

WHAT IS BIOLOGICAL OR FUNCTIONAL DENTISTRY?

Biological dentistry, also known in some circles as holistic dentistry, is the equivalent to functional medicine as its goal is to get to the cause of your oral health issues. It is also termed biocompatible, functional, integrative, biomimetic, or natural dentistry. These names are synonymous and interchangeable. As we now know, thanks to the Harvard Medical School, inflammation is directly linked to the condition in your mouth.

This means that any oral inflammation begets chronic inflammatory mediator release in *all* of your other organ systems. This is a very big deal and is why we are so concerned with any infections that may be present in your mouth.

Biological dentistry deals with:

1. Identifying infections of the teeth, face, bone, glands, soft tissues, and jaws.
2. Understanding heavy metal toxicity and its physiological effects.
3. Knowing how to render damaging and toxic heavy metals inactive by proper removal (IAOMT Protocol).
4. Implementing proper organ meridian identification and teeth-organ connections.
5. Implementing detoxification protocols and detoxification testing procedures.
6. Choosing the best biocompatible replacement dental materials (serum compatibility testing).
7. Understanding the oral inflammatory connection to chronic degenerative disease.
8. Using applicable oral inflammatory disease biomarkers (oral DNA testing).

9. Understanding the role of proper nutrients in oral and systemic CDD.
10. Explaining the periodontal-oral inflammatory and cardiovascular connection.
11. Knowing the functional orthodontic-temporomandibular disorder (TMD) connection.
12. Understanding how to manage acute and chronic oral inflammation (NF-kB).
13. Identifying osteoporosis and its role in oral and gingival-periodontal health.
14. Practicing neuromuscular and functional appliance dentistry.
15. Incorporating dental sleep medicine and obstructive sleep apnea (OSA) into your patient care protocol.
16. Improving the role of immunity by enhancing secretory IgA* function (the NEI-GI oral brain connection).
17. Incorporating and using nutrients that support oral health and bone health.
18. Understanding pH, salivary, GI health and its connection to immune health.
19. Identifying the most biocompatible dental materials for your situation.
20. Using natural methods to maintain oral systemic and gut health (probiotics and S-IgA).
21. Managing pain naturally as a first-line defense to reduce systemic side effects.

In summary, biological dentistry aims to:

- eliminate oral disease.
- restore the oral environment to a healthy function and a healthy state.
- eliminate gingivitis, periodontal disease, oral inflammation, and infection.
- eliminate osteo-cavitations, oral galvanism, and heavy metal toxicity.
- restore proper TMD function and occlusal stability, including neuromuscular function.
- eliminate arch instability and deficiency and restore proper arch form.
- increase masticatory and orthognathic function by increasing the airway space.

* Secretory IgA (SIgA) serves as the first line of defense in protecting the intestinal epithelium from enteric toxins and pathogenic microorganisms. http://www.ncbi.nlm.nih.gov/pmc/articles/PMC3774538/.

The Roots of Health

In health there is freedom. Health is the first of all liberties.
—Henri Frederick Amiel

The suppression of symptoms is taken as a complete solution to medical problems these days. I call it prescription-pad medicine or the Band-Aid approach. Just look at cable TV medical advertising. Integrative medicine and functional dentistry, on the other hand, promote wellness by focusing on the fundamental underlying factors that influence your health. This includes applying solutions that will allow natural healing processes to bring restoration, so that symptoms eventually cease because the underlying causes of the condition are truly addressed.

A friend of mine landed in the hospital for a three-day visit that cost him upward of $17,000 after he'd fallen off a treadmill while exercising at the gym. After three days, I asked him what they had found wrong. He replied, "they really couldn't find anything wrong." I told him that I thought it was most likely an underlying metabolic or nutrient deficit issue or an effect of one of the sleep medications he had been taking. Hospitals don't routinely test for metabolic dysfunction or nutrient levels, because that's not the "standard of care," at least not yet. What they are looking for is the big event—e.g., heart disease, cancer, blockages, etc.

If you have the big event looming on the horizon, they'll probably find it and they may just save your life. But, if it's a metabolic dysfunction or a nutrient deficit they most likely won't find anything wrong. (Good luck with the bill.) So how do we know if we are truly getting sick people well, at the core, instead of just moving symptoms around? And how will we know when they actually become well?

> Functional dentistry and medicine are science-based healthcare approaches that treat illness and promote wellness by focusing on the biochemically unique aspects of each person, and then individually tailoring interventions to restore physiological, psychological, and structural balance.

This approach focuses on understanding the fundamental physiological processes (not alternative processes), the environmental inputs, and the genetic predispositions that influence health and disease so that interventions are focused on treating the cause of the problem, not just masking the symptoms.

Through careful history-taking, symptom questionnaires, and functional laboratory testing, your practitioner can assess fundamental clinical imbalances that may be causing an unhealthy condition. Integrative medicine and dentistry consider multiple factors involved in your health, such as:

- External environmental factors (i.e., toxins)
- Internal neuronal-endocrine imbalances (i.e., aging)
- Disruption of the immune system
- The genetic makeup of the patient (genetic makeup accounts for approximately 5 to 10 percent of disease; genetic SNPs testing is most valuable here)
- Nutrition and lifestyle and metabolic imbalances
- Dental infections and fluctuations in cellular voltage (more about that later)
- Scarring and meridian blockages

Treatment is then designed to address these factors. Often, the correct treatment has to do with how patient lifestyle comes into play and can involve keeping health problems from taking hold in the first place. In that regard, three overarching principles guide the comprehensive, functional approach—sometimes called whole-body treatment—to health:

1. Prevention is paramount and is nutritionally based *and* frequency- and cellular voltage level–based.
2. Integrating whole-body systems and the dynamics of how they function together. I am a systems guy because that is how the Good Lord created us. All the systems are connected, right?
3. You become a partner in your own healthcare. This is most important.

Integrative medicine is also a key to slowing the effects of aging. When root causes of health problems are addressed, the result can be a restoration of youthfulness because the body regains "lost ground."

Age rejuvenation addresses these conditions:

- Weight loss and management
- Perimenopause or menopause
- Toxicity and dental infections, especially failed root canals,* galvanism, and osteo-cavitations
- Thyroid issues and low iodine levels
- Blood sugar issues
- Insomnia and fatigue
- Depression, stress, and anxiety
- Brain fog and candidiasis (overgrowth of candida starts in your mouth and gut)

---

* Scott Laird, ND, and Jodi Laird; Laird Wellness, Root Canals and Breast Cancer, https://rumble.com/v4vs7zb-root-canals-and-breast-cancer.html.

- General preventive medicine and dentistry
- Osteoporosis
- Metabolic syndrome (the real core issue)
- Headaches (often related to food allergies and TMJ problems)

That's why I'm creating a program to address all of these issues. (See the Appendix). But these issues are not confronted by symptom suppression, as in MSM's standard of care. They are addressed through underlying needs of the body, and deeply rooted at the cellular level in our God-given makeup. We're amazingly designed machines, and we're built to run on proper nutrition and voltage, not pharmaceuticals.

BIOLOGICAL SYSTEMS VS. BIOLOGICAL STRESSORS

The Biological Systems

1. Inflammation and the control of NF k-Beta
2. Digestion, detoxification, and the organs of elimination
3. The brain, neurotransmitter balance, and bioenergy voltage
4. The cardiovascular system and mitochondrial support
5. Exocrine and endocrine hormone balancing (BIHRT)
6. Musculoskeletal support system
7. DNA-chromosomal and immune support

The Biological Stressors or Cellular Terrorists

1. Medications such as Dupixent, Toujeo, Jardiance, and many others
2. Aging: your birthday
3. CHOSs, plastic fats, and synthetic foods
4. Stress and anxiety leading to pain
5. Obesity
6. Toxicity, mold, mildew, Epstein-Barr virus (EBV), parasites,* and heavy metals
7. Decreased oxygen metabolism
8. Chronic inflammation and too little oxygen
9. OSA, sleep and breathing disorders
10. Dead water with no mineral load
11. Decreased voltage and frequency
12. Loss of hormones
13. Loss of neurotransmitters, depression, pain (psycho-neuroimmunology)
14. Digestive dysfunction leading to decreased immunity
15. Decreased fulvic and humic acid

* Dr. Lee Merritt, Parasite, Cancer, and Autoimmune Disease, http://www.shelleybholistic nutrition.com/post/dr-lee-merritt-on-parasites-cancer-autoimmune-disease.

16. Mitochondrial energy deficits and overexercising
17. Decreased cell membrane frequency
18. Dental infections and scarring
19. Plastic fatty acids
20. Too much insulin and cortisol
21. Not enough nitic oxide*

The Biological Terrain

The biological terrain consists of factors and conditions needed for proper cellular growth. My friend Dr. Robert Greenberg is a pioneer in biological terrain research, and he brought to my attention this principle that was unknown to me at the time. Think of this terrain like the nutrients existing in the soil that are vital for growing healthy plants. Correct amounts of nutrients and water in soil allow plants to grow healthfully. There is also an organ system called the interstitium or the interstitial fluid. It's known as the ECM or the extracellular matrix, which is the expanse between each cell in your body.

This is the domain of the biological terrain. This ECM is the repository for all nutrients that pass into and out of each one of your cells and is highly governed by the status of the biological terrain.

The oral microbiome and gut microbiome, also termed the gut microbiota, is an integral part of this biological terrain system, contributing to your overall health when it is balanced. When these biological systems are in homeostatic balance, the bugs and disease have a much harder time gaining a foothold.

Similarly, the quality and status of the biological markers in your body—especially your cells—determines how truly healthy you are.

These are some of the biological markers necessary for cellular growth and repair:

- Bodily pH of the blood and in other areas of your body
- Gastric conditions, including the saliva and lymphatic tissue
- Proper enzyme and probiotic level
- Nutrient status or deficiency thereof
- Cellular membrane voltage
- Cofactor levels
- Mineral status
- Proper redox signaling (stands for reduction-oxidation signaling, think electron exchange)
- Water that is biologically sound (i.e., has mineral content, thus has increased voltage)
- Antioxidant levels and cell receptor site sensitivity (this is huge)

* Cardio Miracle, What Is Nitric Oxide, https://cardiomiracle.com/pages/what-is-nitric-oxide.

When was the last time your PCP asked of you any questions related to these topics? Without taking these factors into account, the likelihood of assessing and therefore addressing the body's real needs for improving your health is extremely minimal.

The problem is that these factors are seldom considered thoroughly unless a practitioner is trained in the functional medicine approach to medical problem solving. The effectiveness of any treatment depends on the quality of the patient's *biological terrain* because the terrain is the foundation—the soil—of the body. It also affects the future ability of the body to stave off disease once a patient's health has been stabilized.

So, how do we find out the status of a person's biological terrain so we can know what sort of adjustments are needed in order to bring someone to full health status? Fortunately, a number of evaluation protocols are available.

Here is a list of tests that can be done to prep for functional medicine treatment:

1. Inflammatory cytokine testing
2. Food allergy testing (ALCAT) and bioelectrical impedance analysis (BIA)
3. Candida testing (yeast, SIBO [small intestinal bowel overgrowth])
4. Heart rate variability testing parasympathetic (HRV)—reflects autonomic nervous system (ANS) function absorption and digestive capacity
5. Absorption rate, resistivity, biological terrain testing
6. Oxidative stress testing
7. Mineral testing; spectrox testing
8. Comprehensive digestive stool analysis (CDSA testing)
9. LPP-cardiovascular testing, Apo-B, and oxidized LDL testing
10. CBC panel and serum analysis interpretation
11. Mercury tri-test analysis
12. Salivary hormone analysis
13. Urinary filtrate analysis
14. GTT + Insulin testing
15. Hb-A1c testing, fasting insulin, fasting blood glucose
16. Gastrointestinal dysbiosis analysis
17. Neurotransmitter testing
18. Complete hormone testing (Dutch test)
19. Heavy metals testing, testing for all heavy metals
20. Immuno-genomic testing (SNPSs testing)

Although it's last on the above list, I actually recommend beginning the testing with immuno-genomic testing in order to create a baseline understanding of the patient's biological makeup. Obviously, you'll need professional guidance to know how to proceed with these analyses, but once the biological terrain is understood, then you can go to work on the underlying problems.

Cellular Healing Protocol

Each of the approximately 70 trillion cells (and I'd like to know who's counting these anyway) in your body is a finely tuned machine, designed like a miniature power plant that runs at a specific range of electrical charge. This range for human cells is -20 millivolts (mV) to -25 mV in the cellular membrane. If the cell voltage drops below -20 mV, we become chronically sick or in pain until proper voltage can be restored.*

According to Jerry Tennant, in order to make new cells crucial to ongoing rejuvenation and optimal health, we must achieve a cell-level voltage of -50 mV (an inverse relationship). Voltage flow goes from high voltage to low voltage. This is why you should walk along the beach barefoot, because voltage is higher in the sand along the ocean and flows into your feet, which have lower voltage (that's good), by a process called earthing.†

Additionally, oxygen levels drop when voltage drops, since it is also controlled by the voltage level.‡

When oxygen levels drop, your cells struggle to function properly and cannot produce enough energy in the form of adenosine triphosphate (ATP), in the Krebs cycle. A normal rate of metabolization of fatty-acid molecules, when oxygen levels are normal, is thirty-eight molecules of ATP per one fatty-acid molecule. At lowered oxygen levels, however, ATP production is reduced to as little as two ATP molecules per fatty-acid molecule.§

This is an energy drop of almost 95 percent. This happens in your mitochondria. Think fatigue, fibromyalgia, and cardiovascular issues. It's like a car getting only two miles to the gallon when it's meant to get thirty-eight.

To make matters worse, the trillions of "bugs" that are always in your body but were minding their own business "wake up" when the oxygen level drops, and they go to work producing nasty toxins that negatively affect your health, especially in your failed root canals. They then begin having you for lunch by producing destructive enzymes that dissolve your cells, bones, and connective tissue. As the infected areas housing the toxic enzymes break down, their toxins enter your systemic bloodstream and signal your liver to raise your cytokine inflammatory status, thereby doing more damage. All because of improper voltage and lowered oxygen! The good news, of course, is that restoring correct voltage is very

---

* Jerry Tennant, MD, *Healing Is Voltage* (CreateSpace Independent Publishing Platform; 3rd edition) June 21, 2010.

† Stephen T. Sinatra, MD, *Earthing* (Basic Health Publications, Inc.; 2nd edition).

‡ Tennant, *Healing Is Voltage.*

§ Frank Shallenberger, MD, HMD, *Bursting with Energy* (Basic Health Publications, Inc.).

doable. I've outlined directly below a number of nutritional protocols that can help restore cellular voltage to normal levels.*

- D-Ribose: 10 to 15 mg per day. This supports the formation of ATP in the electron transport cycle. Also take pyrroloquinoline quinone (PQQ), 20 mg a day as this causes mitochondrial biogenesis.
- Essential proper fats, to restore cellular membranes (Nrf2 Renew from Allergy Research Group).†
- Magnesium‡ (Opti You RX): 700 mg per day.
- Humic and fulvic acid, by Allergy Research Group.
- Iodine, by Iodoral: 12.5 mg a day minimum; selenium 800 mcg.
- Testosterone, BIHRT bioidentical hormone replacement therapy, Triiodothyronine, T-3, bioidentical (GTA Forte).
- Concentrace® Trace Mineral Drops§: twenty-one drops per day.
- Pearl Silica Drops®: seven to ten drops per day.
- Sea salt: Take 1 teaspoon, dissolved in one glass of pure water, two times a day.¶
- Lots of veggies. They are electron donors that increase your voltage.
- Hydration through using alkaline water with voltage. People often have decreased mineral content when they are sick and are drinking filtered water. During prolonged illness, drinking water without minerals can dilute your mineral reserve even more, causing a further drop in voltage. This reduction in cellular voltage can make a sick person feel even worse. The answer is to restore the minerals and voltage.
- Increase cholesterol. We'll talk more about modern medical myths later, but one involves cholesterol. All cholesterol-lowering statin drugs are liver toxic and prevent the liver from detoxifying itself, and they reduce coenzyme Q10. But if you clean out the liver by giving it the nutrients it needs to repair itself, your cholesterol will return to a normal and appropriate level, and this will also help to balance hormone function.**
- NT factor: a glycol-phospholipid complex which contains all eight of the nutrients to fix the cell wall (produced by Allergy Research Group).††

---

* Tennant, *Healing Is Voltage*.

† Allergy Research Group, https://www.allergyresearchgroup.com/rf2-renew-120-veget arian -capsules/.

‡ Scott Laird, ND, and Jodi Laird; Laird Wellness; Magnesium, New Research, https://rumble .com/v4m8nez-magnesium-new-researech.html.

§ Concentrace® Trace Mineral Drops; http://www.traceminerals.com.

¶ David Brownstein, MD, *Salt Your Way to Health* (Medical Alternative Press, 2006).

** Stephen T. Sinatra, MD, *The Sinatra Solution, Metabolic Cardiology* (Basic Health Publications, Inc.; Revised, Updated Edition, 2017).

†† All nutraceuticals and supplements mentioned in this book can be ordered on my Dr. Thom 4 Better Health website; http://www.drlokensgard.com/supplements.

- Betaine hydrochloride, called Hydrozyme and made by Biotics Research, Inc. This product helps increase stomach acid for better digestion and the assimilation of nutrients.
- Digestive enzymes. Studies have shown that you heal much faster after surgery when you take digestive enzymes.*
- Probiotics, the more strains the better.
- Prebiotics, fructooligosaccharides (FOS), inulin. All of these support the work of probiotics.
- Sunlight—that's right, you heard me. Twenty minutes a day, without sun block.

So how do you know how much water to drink? The only sure way is to measure intracellular and extracellular fluid levels with a bio-impedance analysis (BIA), but failing that, a valuable rule of thumb is to drink water whenever you feel hungry. The hunger sensation is often the body's signal that it really wants water, not food. So, drink first, then if you still feel hungry, an hour or so after drinking, go ahead and have something to eat. A healthy "standard procedure" is to drink half of your body's weight in ounces every day. For instance, if you weigh 160 pounds, then you'll need to drink 80 ounces of mineralized water each day for optimal hydration. That's 2.5 quarts of water.

Follow the naturopathic principle of CR—caloric restriction (eat less—it's good for you and causes an increase in mitochondria). It's cheaper too. Also, *do not* drink water or anything else before or during a meal, as it will dilute the valuable stomach acid needed to properly digest your protein. "According to Ayurvedic principles, it is generally recommended to maintain a gap of around 45 minutes between food and water intake. Drinking water immediately before or after meals is not advised. However, taking small sips of room-temperature, warm, or hot water during meals is acceptable. Drinking water in large quantities during meals is discouraged. Ayurveda suggests consuming liquids or water in between meals, not before or after eating food.†

To summarize: Chronic disease and pain are always tied to low cellular voltage.‡

So is pain and so is cancer, therefore you've got to raise the voltage to heal the tissue and overcome the chronic problem. Managing pain is simply managing voltage, because pain is a symptom of abnormal voltage. When you smash your thumb with a hammer, according to Dr. Tennant, the voltage immediately is raised to -50 mV and this signals inflammation into the area. It also signals

* A4M, Fellowship in Anti-Aging Regenerative & Functional Medicine; Module III, *Gastroenterology, Neurotransmitters, and Neurology* (Kissimmee, FL, April 2009).

† Life Spa, Ayurvedic Rules About Drinking Water with Meals, https://lifespa.com/diet-detox/hydration/fan-digestive-fire-just-add-water/.

‡ Al Sears, MD, *Confidential Cures Newsletter* (Spring 2008), 1–2.

for healing to occur. When the pain, inflammation, and swelling has fixed your smashed-up thumb, the voltage then returns to -20 mV, and all is well.*

The Secret of Cellular Metabolic Medicine

What happens inside each and every one of our cells is what truly makes the difference so that when I talk about metabolic function, I am referring to metabolism or, loosely put, the burning of oxygen to release energy inside the cell. This generally takes place within the tiny energy factories called mitochondria. These are the "Energizer Bunnies" inside your cells.

After the energy burn, what is left over are compounds called metabolites, which yield essential information about your health condition. We can measure these to see how your cells are operating. However, conventional pharmaceutical-based medicine waits for some big event to happen—a symptom—then applies a medication or surgical intervention to stop the symptom and send you on your way, rather than to "fix" the basic function of the cellular mechanism that led to your big event. To differentiate how prescription-pad (corporate) medicine approaches "cellular" problems versus how cellular metabolic medicine handles these issues, I have outlined several distinctives:

1. Cellular metabolic medicine (CMM) lies outside of the Western traditional allopathic medical prescription pad and disease model, otherwise known as symptom management medicine (my term).
2. In CMM, the hormonal balance, biological terrain, optimization of neurotransmitters, and voltage, are paramount.
3. Diet, breathing, and exercise are the primary therapies that can influence your metabolism, especially omega-3 fatty acids and essential amino acids.
4. The reduction of chronic inflammation is the key to health and can be measured by the markers listed below in the laboratory testing section.

Cellular metabolic medicine measures these markers:

- Alkaline reserves
- Anabolic and catabolic states
- Bio-inflammatory markers
- Bioenergy testing
- Body mass index (BMI)
- Bone index levels

* I highly recommend you read Jerry Tennant's book *Healing Is Voltage* and subscribe to Frank Shallenberger's *2nd Opinion Newsletter.*

- Cardiovascular biomarkers, not just total cholesterol, which has very little to do with heart attacks*
- Digestive inflammatory biomarkers
- Enzyme levels
- Genetic markers and DNA—SNPs markers
- Hormone levels
- Immune modulators
- Key cytokine markers for inflammation
- Metabolic cofactors
- Muscle mass
- Neurotransmitter levels
- Organic acids
- Vitamins and minerals (micro and macro)

With guidance from a knowledgeable practitioner, the results of testing via these markers will help you to formulate a preventive plan that gives you the solutions and products that prevent the bodily rust, disease, and oxidation that can be so deadly.

To summarize, the benefits of cellular metabolic medicine are to:

- Promote nutritional health according to your own personalized needs.
- Address core physiology, not just "alternative" biopharma solutions.
- Improve metabolic functioning at the cellular level, which is to say proper metabolism.
- Integrate and customize health counseling designed for your specific bodily needs.
- Use nutrition and nutraceuticals that strengthen your body and upregulate enzyme systems.
- Detect cellular metabolic problems *before* symptoms occur, even years before.
- Progressively increase your health while decreasing end-stage disease and pain.

Modern Medical and Dental Myopic Myths

Another way to distinguish cellular metabolic medicine from conventional medicine is to show the contrast between the two by looking at what I call the Forty-eight Classic Mainstream Medical and Dental Myopic Myths. They are "myopic" because they reflect a shortsighted way of viewing the body's health needs, mainly for the advertising and sale of products (especially on network television). Scan

* Stephen Sinatra, A4M 18th Annual Congress on Anti-Aging Medicine, conference notes (Orlando, FL, 2010).

through the list below and see how many of these modern myths you still believe. You'll likely be surprised to discover how the "medicalized propaganda" of the past half century has influenced your thinking and may even now make it more difficult to break out of these false ways of thinking about what is and isn't good for you.

Forty-Eight Mainstream Medical and Dental Myths:

1. The **High Salt Diet Is Bad for Me** Myth
2. The **Low-Fat Diet Is Good for Me** Myth
3. The **Fluoride Is Okay for Me and My Children** Myth
4. The **There Is "Truth in Advertising"** Myth
5. The **Cheerios Are Good for Your Heart** Myth
6. The **"Nutrition in Charge" Ensure** Myth (Hint: it's almost all sugar)
7. The **Statin Drugs Are Safe and Cholesterol Is All-Bad** Myth
8. The **Antacids Cure Heartburn** Myth
9. The **Processed Infant Formula Is Okay** Myth
10. The **Bisphosphonates Help My Bones** Myth
11. The **Cholesterol Causes Heart Attacks** Myth
12. The **Saturated Fat Is Bad for Me** Myth
13. The **Vegetable Oils Are Really Good for Me** Myth
14. The **Preprocessed Food Is Just Fine** Myth
15. The **Dairy Products Are Bad for Me** Myth (Hint: raw dairy products are actually good for you; they contain transfer factors.)
16. The **Vegan Diet Contains All the Right Nutrients for Me** Myth (I am a big fan of the mostly plant-based diet. I endorse the "forks over knives diet.")
17. The **I Am Allergic to Iodine** Myth
18. The **I Can Sit on My Butt and Lose Weight** Myth ("The Hollywood Cookie Diet")
19. The **Detoxification Is Not Necessary** Myth
20. The **Digestive Acid Causes Heartburn** Myth (Hint: low acid is usually the problem, called hypochlorhydria.)
21. The **Silver Bullet Can Cure Me** Myth (Hint: your lifestyle is what matters most.)
22. The **It's The Genetics** Myth (Hint: lifestyle again; genetics play a 5 to 10 percent role—maybe.)
23. The **I Need to Count the Calories** Myth (Hint: calories aren't the culprit; it's really insulin signaling.)

24. The **Mercury Fillings Are Okay** Myth
25. The **Nutrition Doesn't Matter** Myth
26. The **My Doctor Has All the Answers** Myth
27. The **My Doctor Says My Labs Are Normal** Myth
28. The **Supplements Are Not Needed** Myth
29. The **Cancer Conundrum** Myth (that we don't know the cause or the treatment for most cancers)
30. The **I Need 60 Percent Carbohydrates** Myth (try 10 percent or less)
31. The **I Can Just Do The "Sensa" Shake to Lose Weight** Myth (I prefer the Hollywood Cookie diet myself.)
32. The **Fat Makes You Fat** Myth (Hint: it's really sugar that makes you fat.)
33. The **USDA Agriculture Food Pyramid Is Good for Me** Myth
34. The **Standard American Diet Is Okay** Myth (it's the exact reverse)
35. The **My Pharmacy Wouldn't Hurt Me** Myth
36. The **Food Industry in No Way Would Ever Hurt Me** Myth
37. The **I Can Just Try Any Diet to Lose Weight** Myth
38. The **Obesity Is a Disease** Myth
39. The **Bottled Water Is Okay for Me** Myth
40. The **FDA Protects the Public** Myth
41. The **My Diet Is Pretty Good** Myth
42. The **My Doctor Knows Best** Myth
43. The **My Insurance Company Cares About Me** Myth
44. The **I Can't Afford to Eat Organic-GMO** Myth (the truth is you can't afford not to)
45. The **Wait Until They Are Done Growing Before We Do Orthodontics** Myth
46. The **Bioidentical Hormones Cause Cancer** Myth
47. The **Vaccines Are Safe and Effective** Myth
    and the biggest travesty of all:
48. The **Government Can Handle Healthcare** Super Myth

It's estimated that 80 percent of the US population is deficient in magnesium and iodine, and I'll talk more later about why this is such a big deal.*

* Jorge Flechas, MD, IAOMT (International Association of Medicine and Toxicology) Annual Spring Meeting, conference notes, 2016.

Remember, also, that lifestyle is responsible for nearly 80 percent of all chronic degenerative disease.*

The reason most doctors simply can't keep up with current medical literature is because medical information doubles every three years or less. Paperwork keeps us preoccupied so we can't keep up with what's really important—red tape, phone calls and ridiculous regulations rule the day. Most of these myths were established in the public consciousness twenty to sixty years ago and now are completely believed by the unsuspecting busy consumer. No wonder we're so sick. Just double-mask and you'll be okay.

* A4M (American Academy for Anti-Aging Medicine) Conference Module 3, conference notes, http://http://www.worldhealth.net.

CHAPTER 2

Total Health Begins in Your Mouth

I saw a TV commercial a while ago that featured a woman talking about having a "smart mouth" of some sort. As I recall, it was an ad about bad breath, and of course, it focused on the awkward social consequences of polluting someone else's personal space with your bad breath. But it got me to thinking: There's a deeper message here. And the message is that your mouth is the window to your body. It is the beginning of your digestive tract, that long, more than twenty-foot tunnel through your body that includes countless crucial bodily functions such as enzymatic functioning to break down foods into amino acids, fatty acids, and carbohydrates, immune detection, metabolic processing, and inflammation control, to name just a few.

Mouthing Off

To start with the bottom-line truth: You cannot have a healthy body without having a healthy mouth. Period. The fact is that total health begins in your mouth. So, what really does that mean? Everything you put into your mouth must be broken down into its amino acid, saccharide, and lipid components (i.e., protein, sugar, and fat). Although this is an amazingly complex process requiring a lot of sequential steps, the really cool thing is that the more you know about the process and how to optimize the way it works for you, the healthier you can become. Of course, you have to do something with what you know.

Knowledge is power, but only knowledge that is acted upon. Remember the discussion about habits and focus, and with regard to health, you *will* see results from the knowledge you act upon.

The metabolic process itself requires prebiotics, probiotics, enzymes, oxygen, proper stomach pH in the form of betaine hydrochloride, cellular signaling, cofactors, iodine, zinc, vitamin B1, thyroid hormone, correct functioning of the nervous system, macro- and micronutrients, minerals, proper mucosal barrier functioning, and lots of energy in the useable form of ATP. Wow, and that's not all. This all depends on oxygen consumption, which is a direct result of the size of your mouth and the airway space it provides. This we refer to as proper airway space. If these systems are not operating at optimum capacity, you may be in trouble and not even know it.*

This is precisely why you need to visit a biological holistic dentistry center. Making sure these systems function properly is our passion because it is so vital to your whole-body health. Period, end of story! Well, actually it's more like the beginning. But you get the picture.

The Heart-Periodontal Link

Periodontal health has been closely tied to vascular health in many studies since the Harvard Medical School first established the connection.† Suboptimal periodontal health occurs when specific types of bacteria proliferate in the gums and mouth, causing imbalanced inflammatory responses. Good oral health has been shown to be linked to optimal cardiovascular function, blood sugar metabolism, and even cognitive health.

Suboptimal periodontal health directly activates inflammatory genetic switches, such as nuclear factor kappa Beta (NF-kB), which negatively impacts endothelial cells in the vessel walls which can interfere with adequate blood-flow to your organs. This is a very big deal, because it affects your microvasculature.

All of the aforementioned inflammatory factors influence the genetic switch, NF-k Beta, that turns on inflammation and regulates nitric oxide and the uptake of oxygen for cellular metabolism.

So, the balance or imbalance of the periodontal-related inflammatory response affects a wide range of critical body systems, including the heart, brain, liver, and kidneys. Therefore, periodontal health is linked to wide-reaching aspects of overall health, and the picture of our health today could well be enhanced simply by improving the health of your mouth.

Current research shows that the mouth has its own unique oral microbiome which directly affects the health of your digestive tract as well. The science behind what I just said is overwhelming. There are two probiotics specifically related to the oral microbiome and upper respiratory tract which will be in our new biological line of dentistry products coming soon.

Bodily Enemy #1: Dental Decay

The number one most common disease in the world is dental decay. The second most prevalent is gingivitis (a reversible, inflammatory condition of your gums), and the third is periodontal disease. And if your dentistry team has diagnosed inflammation in your mouth, you also have unchecked chronic inflammation in

---

* Tennant, *Healing Is Voltage*, et al.

† Harvard Medical School, "Treating gum disease may lessen the burden of heart disease, diabetes, other conditions." Heart Health, 2014. http://www.health.harvard.edu/blog/treating-gum-disease-may-lessen-burden-heart-disease-diabetes-conditions-201407237293.

your body. This can lead to a myriad of unhealthy, nagging symptoms, generalized chronic inflammation, such as:

- chronic pain and inflammation
- fatigue
- headaches
- digestive issues
- bad breath
- weight gain
- memory loss
- gas
- bloating
- anxiety

Any or all of these can signal the beginning of more serious health conditions such as:*

- candidiasis
- cardiovascular disease
- stroke
- diabetes
- accelerated aging
- hormonal and neurotransmitter imbalances
- hypertension
- pancreatic and other cancers
- osteoporosis
- low-birth-weight babies
- toxicity

The good news is that all of these can be improved—and sometimes reversed—or slowed by making the sort of healthy lifestyle changes we're talking about in this book. And you can start by cleaning the window—your mouth—by understanding the basics of a healthy lifestyle, proper oral care, and eating habits.

Since we're focusing on the influence of your mouth on your health, it's important to know which dentistry problems can cause most of your health-related issues. Probably the biggest concerns that relate directly to your mouth are heavy metal toxicity and dental infections, but there are several more. Let's first take a look at toxicity because the number and size of mercury fillings in your mouth are directly related to the amount of mercury in your brain which can cross into placental tissue (a serious problem for pregnancy). The fact is that there

* American Dental Association, (ADA), Oral-Systemic Health, ADA Science & Research Institute, https://www.ada.org/resources/ada-library/oral-health-topics/oral-systemic-health/.

is no safe level of mercury in the body. The presence of mercury is like a dripping faucet that, little by little, accumulates to a tipping point called the Total Body Burden. This is the point at which the toxicity begins to cause noticeable problems, and it's different for each individual.*

So you'll know how serious the problem of amalgam fillings actually is, consider a couple of comparisons. A fluorescent light bulb—which we all recognize contains toxic gas—encloses about 20 mg of mercury in a four-foot-long tube. A more compact bulb holds about 6 mg. By comparison: A large molar filling contains 750 mg to 1,000 mg of mercury. That's enough to contaminate a five-acre lake so that it wouldn't be safe to eat the fish caught there. Mercury is also highly suspected to contribute to autism.†

Mercury depletes intracellular glutathione, which reduces your intracellular ability to detoxify. Tylenol, (or any acetaminophen product) also lowers glutathione production, thereby limiting your ability to detoxify intracellularly. Stay far away from and never use acetaminophen for anything.

Millions of people, of course, have mercury fillings in their mouths, and it would be nice to simply say, "They should have them removed." While that would be ideal, the removal process is not something to be taken lightly. When mercury fillings are *not* removed correctly, the process can actually make matters worse. If not done correctly, filling removal disperses toxic methylated mercury vapors, which both patient and practitioner ingest. Inhaling of the vapors moves mercury directly into the body and allows it to cross the blood-brain barrier. It then lodges in the brain and, in pregnant women, in the placenta and the unborn.‡

The continued use of mercury fillings seems almost inexcusable. It has been banned in most European and South American countries. Mercury was first used for fillings as long ago as the 1830s—at a time when treatment of diseases with mercury taken internally was still considered the "standard of care." A typical amalgam filling is about half mercury. The rest is a combination of other metals such as copper, tin, zinc, gold, and silver. In our office, we never place these mercury fillings, although in traditional dentistry, about 30 percent of dentists still use these toxic fillings, including pediatric dentistry where they are placing mercury next to the blood-brain barrier. That is why we call them mercury fillings. Any wonder why autism has increased tremendously over the past fifty years?§, ¶

---

* Holistic Dental Association (HDA); International Academy for Biological Dental Medicine (IABDM);International Association of Medicine and Toxicology (IAOMT), various conference notes.

† *Vaxxed, The Film They Don't Want You To See* (director, Dr. Andrew Wakefield, producer, Del Bigtree) https://vaxxedthemovie.com/.

‡ American Academy for Anti-Aging Medicine (A4M); HAD; The Institute for Functional Medicine (IFM) IABDM; IAOMT, et al.

§ *Vaxxed, The Film They Don't Want You To See.*

¶ Del Bigtree, *Vaxxed: Pulling Back the Curtain*; the Highwire, https://thehighwire.com/ark-videos/episode-64-vaxxed-pulling-back-the-curtain.

As mercury builds up in your system, these are the factors that affect how your body will cope:

1. Are you excreting it via a properly functioning liver?
2. Are your kidneys performing as they should?
3. Are you constipated?
4. Are you also iodine deficient?
5. Where do you live—near coal-fired power plants or waste dumps?
6. What are the other sources of mercury that you consume?
7. Do you have fibromyalgia, chronic fatigue syndrome (CFS), or decreased mitochondrial function?

Heavy metal toxicity is one of the issues in dental health that can affect the entire body. Here is a rundown on the other problems.

The next most debilitating conditions in my opinion are:

- **Failed Root Canals and Dental Infections.*** These must be addressed and removed properly! Dental infections and abscessed areas in your jaws release toxic substances into your systemic circulation every time you chew or bite down, thus resulting in an inflammatory cascade of cytokine modulators that trigger a compound in your liver called hs-CRP. Left unchecked, this increases the inflammatory process and causes the inflammation to become chronic. You then move into chronic overdrive if the situation is not dealt with. You would most likely be unaware of this problem unless pain is involved.†

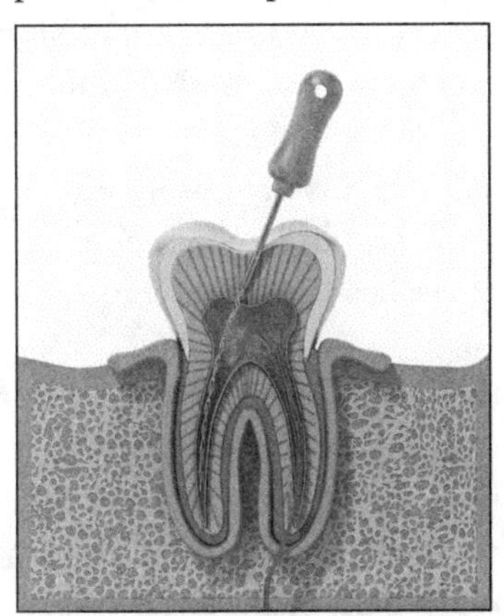

3-D illustration of root canal treatment process. Credit: adventtr.

* *The Root Cause*, directed by Frazer Bailey, starring Ben Purser; the documentary has been banned on most sources, but can be viewed at https://tubitv.com/movies/507721/root-cause.

† DAMS (Dental Amalgam Mercury Solutions) http://http://www.amalgam.org; HDA; IABDM; IAOMT, et al.

- **Your inability to chew** and completely pulverize your food has a direct correlation as to how well you absorb nutrients in your gut. (While some people say "you are what you eat," I say "you are what you absorb.")
- **Root canals and the related meridian blockages** of certain organs can become a serious problem.
- **TMJ problems** can contribute to headaches, jaw opening, and facial issues.
- **Galvanic currents** can cause hearing imbalances, ringing in the ears, and improper voltage in the cell membrane, thus causing healing delays.
- **Periodontal disease** can cause cardiovascular problems as well as some cancers, low birth weight in babies, and can contribute to dementia.
- **Implants** can interfere with acupuncture meridians and cause issues in the jaws unless properly placed. I believe that ceramic implants are superior to titanium implants and are the best replacement, today, for infected failed root canals. Just make sure that you have the extracted tooth sockets replaced with PRF and ozone, plus have the periodontal ligaments removed during the extraction process.
- There is a procedure called **Auto-Hemolytic Therapy or 10-Pass**, which is ozone injected into your venous system, thereby raising nitric oxide[*] levels in your endothelium. NO levels are critical to keep at a high functioning level.[†]
- The **size and opening of your airway space**, along with tongue size, can contribute to sleep, snoring, OSA, and breathing issues. It can also contribute to poor metabolism which can cause fatigue. You must always evaluate tongue-ties and arch space, then have them properly diagnosed.
- **Osteo-cavitations** can be caused by improper tooth extractions and failed root canals and can trigger a myriad of misdiagnosed jaw and health issues.
- **Microbial biofilm** that remains in your mouth needs to be addressed and removed—especially porphyromonas gingivalis and mercury in the brain, both of which have been implicated in Alzheimer's disease.[‡]

The Dentinal Fluid Transport System (DFTS)

Ralph Steinman and John Leonora have done a tremendous amount of research on the DFTS, which remains largely ignored by most others. For years, dentistry has been trying to figure out why some people get rampant decay and others pay no attention to their oral care or diet, yet rarely, if ever, experience dental decay.

---

* http://www.CardioMiracle.com.

† Nathan Bryan, PhD, and Janet Z and, OMD, *The Nitric Oxide (NO) Solution* (Neogenesis, 2010).

‡ Thomas J. Lewis, PhD, and Clement L. Trempe, MD. *The End of Alzheimer's; The Brain and Beyond* (Academic Press, 2017).

Part of the answer centers on what happens in the "hydraulic-pump" system of the DFTS. The flow of fluids in and out of the teeth can cause or reduce decay.*

Each one of your teeth contains miles of microscopic, micro-tubular super highways called odontoblastic dentinal tubules. These little tubules make up the dentinal fluid transport system (DFTS), which is responsible for carrying enzymes, minerals, amino acids, and other critical substances into and out of your teeth. The way this system operates depends on several components and concepts.

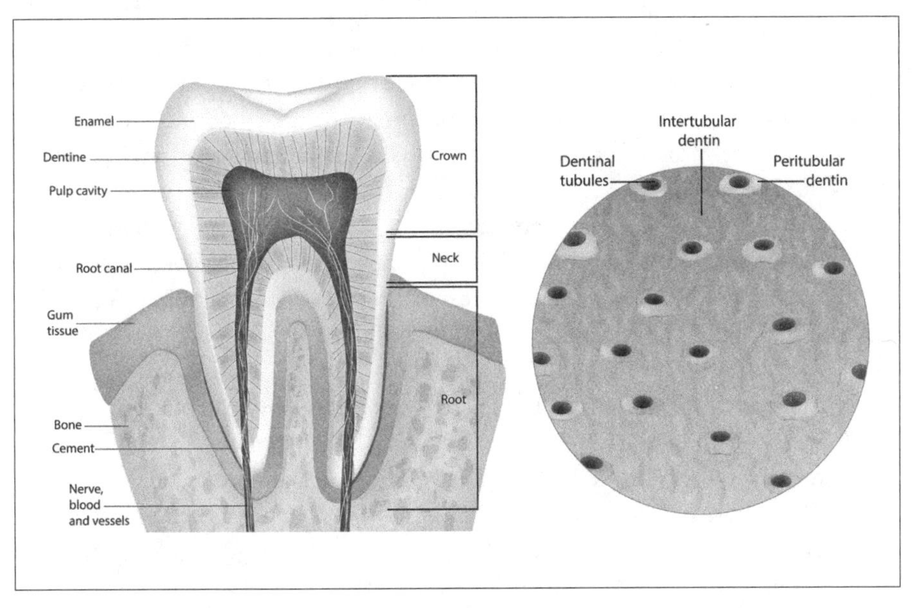

Dentin or dentine structure. Intertubular dentin, peritubular dentin, dentinal tubules. Cross-section of the layers of teeth. Credit: Sakurra.

Dental Fluid Transport System (DFTS). This is an overall depiction of the DFTS. The microtubular channels are responsible for nourishing your teeth. They also contribute to the sensitivity after a tooth has had a filling or crown procedure.

The closer to the pulp you get, the more tubules there are, and the bigger in diameter they become. This is a highly valuable, necessary, and overlooked system that plays a huge role in how your teeth and body function and whether or not they remain healthy. It is the center of the body's process for remineralization or demineralization (osteoblastic vs. osteoclastic balance) of the teeth matrices.

The way this works is complex, but I've outlined below the key concepts about how the system operates. Follow me here as (Dr. Roggenkamp, a student

* Clyde Roggenkamp, DDS, MSD, MPH, *Dentinal Fluid Transport* (Loma Linda University Press, October 31, 2005).

of Steinman and Lenora, wrote an entire book on their research, which I've simplified and summarized for you.):*

1. Dentin is living tissue, composed of cells called odontoblasts. They are dependent on a bidirectional transport system that has no vascular blood supply. It runs on dentinal lymph fluid (DLF).
2. Dentinal lymph fluid is designed for transport in the direction from the dental pulp to the enamel interface. The enamel is also porous, so it facilitates fluid flow to the outside of the tooth. A hydrostatic pressure gradient exists in the system and favors the flow of nutrients from inside the pulp chamber to the enamel surface on the outside of the tooth.
3. The DFTS is driven by the hypothalamic-parotid endocrine axis. (Let's call it the HPEA, for short, okay?) This is the signaling pathway for the fluid transport.
4. The DFTS is a pump system in which the fluid in the pulp chamber is derived from the blood. The fluid pumped through the tubular system is composed of blood proteins, minus the large blood protein molecules. It's called dental lymph fluid, and it contains essential nutrients for maintaining the vitality of the dentin.
5. The essential nutrients in the dental lymph fluid are: glucose for metabolism, amino acids for synthesizing dentinal collagen, and minerals (including silica) to mineralize the dentinal collagen.
6. This whole system is dependent on proper pH. You must maintain consistent acid levels above 6.0—this is why alkaline diets along with alkaline oral health products are so important.
7. This transport system is also dependent on a hormone from the parotid gland called the parotid hormone, which is signaled by the pituitary gland in the brain.
8. In healthy teeth, the fluid flow direction is outward toward the enamel surface from the pulpal chamber which is inside the tooth.
9. The hydrostatic pressure within the teeth is higher than in the mouth, and this differential causes the odontoblastic cells to pump fluid from inside the pulp to the enamel surface (the correct direction for the process of remineralization).
10. In decayed, unhealthy teeth, this fluid flow is reversed—a major-league big deal. Flow in the wrong direction allows oral fluids to gain entrance into the dentin through the enamel and cause cariogenesis—i.e., tooth decay.

---

* Roggenkamp, *Dentinal Fluid Transport.*

Now, let me summarize how they work together:

The parotid gland. This is the major salivary gland on the inside of your cheeks that is responsible for salivary production. It's also responsible for the relay signaling from the hypothalamus, which in turn, drives the system.

The hypothalamus is the master gland in your brain responsible for signaling and relaying to the parotid gland the production of parotid hormone.

The parotid hormone (PH). This hormone alters the permeability of the odontoblastic cell membrane. Herein lies the key. It allows for the unwanted inward flow of dental lymph fluid into the odontoblasts. These are the cells that make dentin, sometimes called dentine. The pH then enters the circulation and activates the DLF present in the odontoblasts.

The **dentinal lymph fluid (DLF)** has a great ability to buffer the pH of the fluid at 7.4, and to keep this fluid pH at the same level as the blood. Again, you can see the importance of proper pH. If it's too low, the proper functioning of this critical system is disrupted.

The acidic environment of high-sugar diets reverses the flow of the DFTS. Sugar suppresses the function of the HPEA and leads to a decrease in pH secretion. This shuts down the normal functioning of the DFTS.

The sucrose effect. Diets high in sucrose (processed sugar) inhibit the production and flow of saliva and have been shown to cause atrophy of the parotid glands. This also decreases the alkaline environment, thus favoring tooth decay.

The effect of endogenous compounds. Certain compounds like carbamoyl aspartate and carbamoyl phosphate,* which is in our new toothpaste, cause proper mineral flow that can reduce the rate of caries by nearly 90 percent.

Bodily Enemy #2 Gingivitis and #3 Periodontal Disease

I said at the beginning of this chapter that gingivitis is the second most common disease in the world. But what, exactly, is it? Simply put, gingivitis is inflammation of the gum tissue caused by an unchecked bacterial biofilm, manifested as a red, swollen condition of the gums. Fortunately, the malady is reversible, if treated effectively and early. I can't overstate the importance of early and effective treatment, though, because if not addressed, gingivitis can lead to bodily enemy #3, periodontal disease, which is not reversible. Periodontal disease causes loss of bone and gum tissue which cannot be replaced.

---

* Pearl Nature's Toothpaste has this special ingredient, http://www.PearlOralHealth.com.

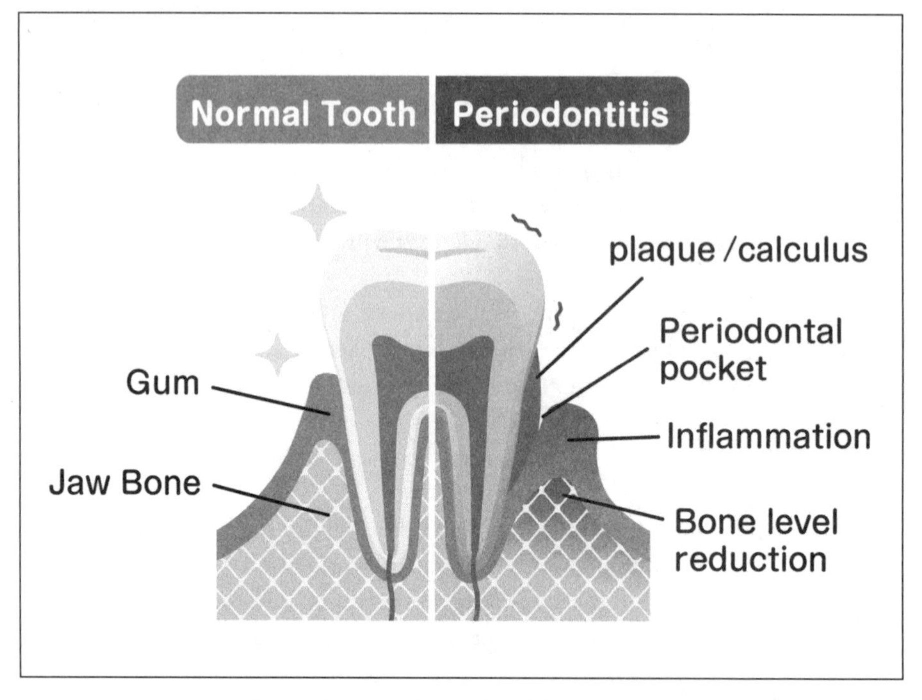

Comparison of normal teeth and periodontal disease. Credit: Barks_japan.

As a result, periodontal disease can lead to several serious problems:

- Chronically infected gums
- Tooth and bone loss
- Elevation of chronic inflammatory biomarkers
- Increased heart disease and stroke incidence

Periodontal disease is also one of the most significant indicators and determinants of whole-body health. The elevation of inflammatory biomarkers is the beginning of cardiovascular and chronic degenerative disease. Obviously, this is really bad news.*

The good news, though, is what you can do to prevent the cascading effects of gingivitis and periodontal disease. This simple statement in a report about gum disease by BBC News World Edition on November 26, 2002, captures the essence of your battle plan: "Antioxidants fight off gum disease."

Why is this?

People with severe gum disease have been found to have low levels of antioxidant chemicals that, if present, may offer natural protection. Other studies have shown that periodontal disease appears to be a genuine threat to general health. It

* Thomas E. Levy, MD, JD, *Hidden Epidemic* (Medfox Publishing, 2017), 160–62.

is not only the primary cause of teeth loosening but has been linked to both the onset of diabetes and the worsening of lung disease.*

Recent studies have even pointed to gum disease as a potential threat to unborn children. The University of Birmingham (England) school of dentistry may have perhaps found a clue as to why. After analyzing the type of saliva called gingival crevicular fluid, researchers found that this key salivary component had a much higher level of an intracellular antioxidant called glutathione in patients with healthy gums. Dr. Simon Langley-Evans, a nutritional lecturer at Nottingham University, told the BBC that if you have periodontal disease, the first thing you should do is stop smoking.† Cigarette smoke destroys antioxidants.

Glutathione appears to be a key antioxidant that could be a predictor for periodontal disease.

Untreated, the damage happens this way: your gum tissue hugs your tooth like a turtleneck sweater hugs your neck. If the hygienist can probe more than three millimeters past the top of the gum margin, then it indicates a periodontal condition. Other unwanted bugs can get inside the "turtleneck" and cause problems. The turtleneck is a barrier to your systemic circulation also known as the gingival sulcus barrier.

The Alzheimer's Disease Connection

Because the tragic condition of Alzheimer's disease is so common these days, it's worth noting, in particular, the disturbing connection between periodontal problems and Alzheimer's disease. Bacteria in your blood seems to be a factor, and the most suspicious culprit is *Porphyromonas gingivalis* (Pg). And guess where that comes from? Pg is a bacterial species present in the gum tissue of those who have gingivitis. And the Alzheimer's disease connection? According to the *Journal of Alzheimer's Disease*,‡ *P. gingivalis* was found in the brains of four out of ten samples of brain tissue in patients who exhibited Alzheimer's disease. The clear implication is that bacteria from the mouth can enter the bloodstream through chewing and cleaning by entering the gingival sulcus barrier and ending up in other parts of the body, including your brain. In his May 10, 2013, article, Dr. St. John Crean§ points to a solution: "the issue is to reduce the bacterial load that

---

* Levy et al., *Hidden Epidemic*, 52, 62.

† Dr. Simon Langley-Evans, "Antioxidants Fight off Gum Disease," http://news.bbc.co.uk/2/hi/health/2512357.stm.

‡ *Journal of Alzheimer's Disease* (JAD), "New Study Reveals an Association Between the Presence of Certain Infections and Later Development of Alzheimer's Disease." https://www.j-alz.com/content/new-study-reveals-association-between-presence-certain-infections-and-later-development.

§ Professor St. John Crean, Dean of School of Medical and Dentistry, University of Central Lancashire, http://www.aesthet icdentalsolutions.co.uk/meet-us/lytham/prof-st-john-crean-oral-maxillofacial-services-lytham/; Gum Health Link, https://www.aestheticdentalsolutions.co.uk/news/.

occupies our gum tissues, to reduce the bacterial assault." That means you need to address periodontal disease and gingivitis for the sake of your overall health and to reduce your chances of succumbing to Alzheimer's disease. The starting point is to ask your dentistry team for a periodontal probing and gingivitis examination.

Another potential culprit in the Alzheimer's connection also has dental roots (so to speak). Heavy metals, especially mercury and aluminum, have been implicated in many neurological diseases, including Alzheimer's disease. Mercury, as we've discussed, is all too present in traditional amalgam fillings, and aluminum is a surreptitious ingredient in vaccines, many cosmetic and bakery products (another reason you need to read labels on everything you buy). Thanks FDA, for keeping us safe, and at such a reasonable cost.

Natural Prevention and Healing of Gingivitis and Periodontal Disease

Chronic inflammation, which contributes to 80 percent of the known chronic degenerative disease conditions, is largely caused by lifestyle. Although genetics can play a role, it usually is far less of a factor than lifestyle. Keeping your teeth, gums, and periodontal tissues inflammation-free is not just an option for good health, it's a *must* to prevent the insidious onset of many diseases. Fortunately, there's a lot you can do to keep your mouth healthy.

I've outlined below some of the most significant and doable things you can work into your daily regimen.

To maintain healthy gums, teeth, and periodontal tissues:

- **Take iodine.** (Iodoral, Povidine Iodine, or Lugol's). This helps alkalinize your oral tissues, which is a protocol to prevent decay and periodontal disease. I recommend a minimum of 12.5 mg per day.
- **Apply Argentyn 23®** (silver hydrosol).* Four times a day, hold it under your tongue, then swallow. Argentyn 23® is an antibiotic that is also a highly effective antibacterial, antiviral, antifungal, and antiprotozoal.
- **Oil pulling,**† To remove toxins, cure tooth decay, prevent cavities, whiten teeth, heal bleeding gums, and improve breath, use 1 tablespoon of coconut oil as a mouth rinse once per day. Start by swishing for two to three minutes, working up to ten to twenty minutes per day, then spit into the trash as it may clog your drain. Don't swallow.
- **Swish and rinse with Celtic sea salt, Bob's Red Mill salt, or Himalayan pink salt**. You can take 1 teaspoon of "unrefined" sea salt up to three times per day, mixed with water. This increases cellular

* Immunogenics Corporation (Sarasota, FL) https://naturalimmunogenics.com/.

† Sahara Rose Ketabi, *Ayurveda*, (Alpha/Penguin Random House, LLC, 2017), 142–143.

membrane voltage, which needs to be between -20 mVs to -25 mVs, and also lowers blood pressure.*

- **Probiotic therapy** will help alkalinize your biofilm (see my probiotic instructions in the appendix).
- **Pearl Silica Drops®**† Adults take six to ten drops (children, three to five drops) of absorbable silica daily in water or juice. This product is highly alkalinizing and remineralizing.
- Drink **purified, mineralized water.**
- **Use a Sonicare**, a sonic toothbrush that effectively removes plaque, rather than a manual toothbrush. It is better at destroying bacteria and it reaches below the gumline.
- **Use a tongue scraper** first thing in the morning, then apply coconut or ozone oil. (Tongue scraping is the practice of gently grazing the tongue with the help of a u-shaped tool or a scraper to remove the debris and bad bacteria from the surface of the tongue‡)
- **Do not use a commercial mouth rinse.** It kills beneficial bacteria.
- **Grape seed extract,**§ which is loaded with antioxidants that will kill *H. pylori*¶ in the gut and raise nitric oxide levels.**
- **Xylitol gum decreases** *Streptococcus mutans* and *Streptococcus pneumoniae*, the same bacteria that cause dental decay and middle ear infections, respectively. Discovered more than a century ago, xylitol has been scrutinized in more than 1,500 scientific studies. In a number of clinical trials, this natural sweetener has been shown to reduce plaque formation and inhibit streptococcus mutans, the bacteria primarily responsible for causing cavities, tooth decay, and gum disease.†† Do not give xylitol to your pets. They cannot digest this type of sugar, and it could be fatal.
- **Nutritional therapy, especially coenzyme Q10** and by following the alkaline food list.

---

* Scott Laird, ND, and Jodi Laird; Laird Wellness; Salt and Blood Pressure, https://rumble.com/v49cako-salt-and-blood-pressure.html. Do check with your trusted health care professional if you are suffering from kidney disease before starting this regimen.

† Pearl Oral Health, http://www.PearlOralHealth.com.

‡ Ayurveda: The Benefits of Tongue Scraping, https://artoflivingretreatcenter.org/blog/ayurveda-101-the-benefits-of-tongue-scraping/.

§ Pearl Nature's Toothpaste has this special ingredient, http://www.PearlOralHealth.com.

¶ Jose Manuel Silvan et. al., *Pre-Treatment with Grape Seed Extract Reduces Inflammatory Response and Oxidative Stress Induced by Helicobacter pylori Infection in Human Gastric Epithelial Cells*, http://www.mdpi.com/2076–3921/10/6/943.

** Nathan Bryan, PhD, and Janet Zand, OMD, *The Nitric Oxide (NO) Solution* (Neogenis 2010).

†† Rallie McCallister, MD, *The Benefits of Xylitol* (white paper).

- **Use the twelve compounds that control bad breath** (see the next section and follow the list).
- **Floss, floss, and floss** or use periodontal aids or both.
- **Avoid refined sugar.** (Find appropriate substitutes in my Safe Sugars List.)
- **Balance your pH** by alkalinizing your biofilm with lemon water or ConcenTrace Liquimins. Swish or rinse with water, after meals and any snacks. This dilutes the oral acid content.
- **Use Pearl Nature's Toothpaste®** at least twice a day.

If you have been diagnosed with periodontal disease, then you need to get serious about a treatment plan that consists of daily management of your periodontal pockets and the elimination of the bleeding in your gums. This is serious business that you need to control daily.

What Causes Bad Breath?

Foul breath is caused by a bacterial breakdown product that releases sulfur gas in the mouth. This methyl mercaptan compound is released when excessive bacterial toxins, periodontal disease, or gingivitis are present. These are the various triggers for the conditions that create bad breath:

- **Periodontal disease.** Contributes greatly to the excess buildup of sulfur groups produced by endotoxins that live below the gumline. They live in a medium called the gingival crevicular fluid, which can harbor billions of gas-producing bacteria and spirochete organisms.
- **Bacteria embedded in your tongue.** To avoid this cause, use a tongue scraper to clean the top surface of your tongue.
- **Excessive dry mouth.** Many medications and some cancers contribute to this issue. Check a PDR for the drugs you are taking.
- **Esophageal gastric reflux and bacterial toxins from stomach problems.** Answer: Increase your stomach acid. This is a tried-and-true naturopathic principle. You can use Hydrozyme®, from Biotics Research®.
- **Bacterial toxins in your sinuses** that turn chronic. This includes bacteria but especially yeast and fungus that produce methyl mercaptan. Use OxyMist®,[*] which is hypochlorous acid (HOCL) and is antibacterial, antifungal, and antiviral or Argentyn-23® (also known as Sovereign Silver).[†]

---

[*] Pearl Oral Health, https://pearloralhealth.com/.

[†] Seth Quinto, CEO Immunogenics Corporation (Sarasota, Florida) https://naturalimmunogenics.com/.

If you pay attention to TV commercials, you would think that the perfect solution to bad breath is to use the "right mouthwash." A swish a day, and your problem is solved, right? Way wrong. As you know by now, that is a purely superficial solution to a complex issue. Many Big Pharma mouth-rinse formulations are toxic. Fortunately though, the real solution is not difficult, either, and many of the "answers" even taste good. For starters, here's a list of foods and drinks that can help get to the root of a bad breath problem:

1. Alkaline or ozonated water
2. Apples
3. Green tea (contains EGCG)
4. Cherries
5. Parsley (contains polyphenols)
6. Whole, raw milk
7. Spinach (more polyphenols); eat it raw to maintain the lutein levels
8. Lettuce
9. Spearmint (contains chlorophyll)
10. Basil
11. Citrus fruits (eat between meals as snacks; do not eat with protein)
12. Yogurt with probiotics, especially *Streptococcus thermophilus* and *Lactobacillus bulgaricus*

Be careful with yogurt. It's mostly sugar. The best I've found is Stonyfield Organic Plain. Good dental hygiene practices will help reduce bad breath as well. It's crucial to brush, floss, and rinse frequently to minimize the bacterial toxic load. I recommend the following to really round out your bad breath treatment:

- Argentyn-23®, a nanotech, silver-hydrosol antibiotic, antiviral, and antifungal product which is highly effective with no downside risk. It's also an immune booster. (Available from Natural Immunogenics.)*
- Take a multi-strain probiotic. This is very effective in combating unfriendly bacteria. (Ancient Nutrition has a line of SBO probiotics.)
- Neutralizing the acidity in your mouth with alkalinizing water and/or sea salt, or baking soda, are good ideas. Your oral pH should be around 6.5 to 7.0 in the morning. Test with pH strips.
- Reduction of refined sugars is a must because bacteria and cancer feed on sugar. (Follow the Weston A. Price Foundation and Price-Pottenger Nutritional Foundation protocols on this one.)†

* https://naturalimmunogenics.com/.

† Weston A Price Foundation, (WAPF) http://www.westonaprice.org; Price-Pottenger Nutrition Foundation, (PPNF) https://price-pottenger.org/.

- Chew xylitol gum.
- OxyMist® is an all-natural, topical facial and skin spray product from Pearl Oral Health* which is antibacterial, antiviral, and antifungal.

So, now that you are alerted to the importance of good oral health as an indicator and determinant of your overall health, what can you do to optimize the well-being of your mouth? I'm glad you asked because that's exactly what I plan to address in chapter 3.

* http://http://www.PearlOralHealth.com.

CHAPTER 3

Making Your Mouth Healthy Again

As we age, various organ systems begin to "pause" or change in functionality. Dr. Eric Braverman recognized this pattern and delivered to medical science a brilliant understanding of how aging impacts the organs of our bodies and how they function. Realizing the value of his approach, I decided there must be an application of this "pause principle" to oral health, and I've found that, in fact, a clear understanding of that principle is the necessary foundation to developing optimal oral health at any stage of life.*

The Oral Pauses of Life Medical Model

A look at our external features offers a clue as to what is going on inside us as we age. Aging oral pauses affect your mouth and your face. In fact, there are fourteen distinct dentally oriented pauses that I have identified:

1. Periopause
2. Enamopause
3. Salivopause
4. Gingivopause
5. Osteopause
6. Dentopause
7. Dentinopause
8. Lipopause
9. Cementopause
10. Somatopause
11. Adipopause
12. Faciopause
13. Collagenopause
14. Dermatopause

* Eric R. Braverman, MD, *The Healing Nutrients Within: Facts, Findings, and New Research on Amino Acids* (Basic Health Publications, Inc.; 3rd ed., 2012), 169–72.

That's a lot of pausing in your mouth and face. Although each pause affects a specific aspect of your oral and facial function, the common problem identified by the pause model is that, as we age organs, cells, and their associated systems begin to shut down. Remember, you have to focus on systems. Whole-body systems. The relay systems that establish normal function and govern production and distribution of hormones, neurotransmitters, and genetic proteins change over time and are involved in cellular senescence, also known as cellular death, or apoptosis.*

So, what drives these changes in the mouth and face? At this point, you might not be surprised to learn that the cause for the pause is silent inflammation and lowered metabolism. The fourteen pauses I've outlined above are the inflammatory changes that occur at or above your neck.

To understand how we can address the inflammatory pauses in your mouth, we need to look at several important components and issues in oral functioning: saliva, lymphatics, urinary filtrate, and osteo-cavitations.

Saliva and Its Function

Saliva does a lot more for your body than simply keep your mouth from feeling dry. As with other aspects of your oral functioning, it reflects crucial aspects of your overall health, and we can begin to grasp why by understanding the basics about saliva.

Your saliva is made up of three components: two proteins and one fluid. The serous portion of saliva contains the compounds hyaline and alpha amylase, a salivary protein. The other protein, a mucin protein, helps with lubrication and hydration of your food. These are contained within a fluid base called the interstitial fluid or sometimes referred to as the interstitial matrix. The fluid is produced by the acinar cells and delivered to the mouth through the interlobular duct.

The content of saliva is a good representation of the lymphatic system and your digestive capability. Why? Because, by examining and testing saliva we can also see what's going on with oxidation in the lymphatic system (ZRT salivary testing). This can reveal valuable information regarding your overall health. Acinar cells, for example. are located in the pancreas as well as the mouth.

As a result, from what is happening in the mouth, we can draw some conclusions as to what may be happening in the pancreas. Saliva also tells us about the lymphatic tissue and the status of the small intestine.†

* Life Extension, The Science of a Healthier Life, *Combat Aging by Reducing Senescence Cell Burden*, by Sean Field (Winter Ed, 2019-2020) 14-19.

† ZRT Laboratory Testing Manual, http://www.zrtlab.com/.

The Lymph Connection

Your lymph system is a critical producer of antioxidants—the means by which your body reduces the presence of free radicals. While two thirds of your lymphatic tissue production occurs in the liver and the cells surrounding the small intestine (its interstitial cells), the remaining third of this essential tissue is made in the salivary acinar cells.

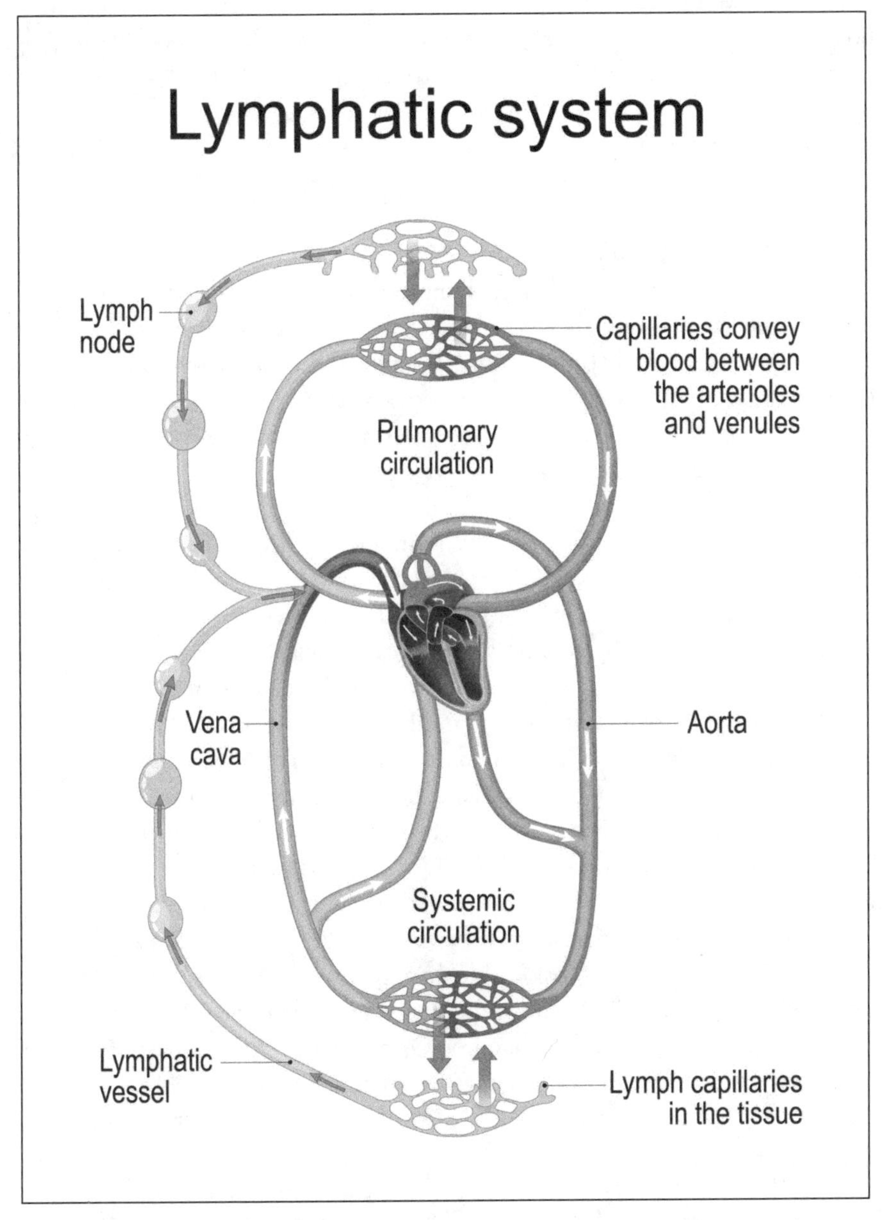

Lymphatic circulation system, lymph node, blood vessel, capillaries, and heart. Credit: ttsz.

"This is why saliva can tell us about liver tissue, the small intestine, and pancreatic activity, and is why you must do more than bloodwork."[*, †]

If you can measure the oxidative stress of lymphatic tissue, then you have a good measure of the antioxidant production of the liver, pancreas, and the overall gastrointestinal tract. When the saliva is analyzed, it is possible to determine the level of antioxidant production and, hence, the functionality of these organs. In addition, we can find out about carbohydrate metabolism in the mouth and the pancreas, a crucial factor in the digestive process. It's also possible to judge the production and balance of sex hormones required for normal whole-body functioning.[‡]

Amazing what you can find in your mouth. See chapter 1 for the lists of tests you can do these days on your own or with your practitioner's help.

The Problem with Osteo-Cavitations

Osteo-cavitations, or areas of dead bone, are also called NICO lesions. This stands for neuralgia-inducing cavitational osteonecrosis. These lesions are hollow places in your jawbones. Interestingly, though, the concept of jawbone cavitation is controversial. Many dental professionals refuse to believe that these bony lesions even exist. However, in the specialties of orthopedics, neurosurgery, and internal medicine, these lesions are well-recognized.

Many lie dormant and are quite painless, often for decades. Yet the reality is that these despicable intrusions are like a smoldering fire which can blaze to life under certain conditions. It is estimated, for instance, that at least 20 percent of all hip replacements in the United States are due to osteonecrosis.

NICO lesions have been described as a cavity within a cavity. (I like to call them "just another hole in your head that you don't know about.")

The effect of these lesions in the mandible (lower jaw) and the maxilla (upper jaw) are similar because both are medullary bones. This means they each have bone marrow and produce blood cells, and it is usually within these medullary spaces that cavitations occur. Blockages in tiny blood vessels reduce blood flow, thus robbing oxygen from areas of the bone and ultimately causing bone death called necrosis. The process is similar to a stroke.[§]

The diagnosis of cavitations can be hindered by the fact that they are not always obvious on X-rays. Considerable diagnostic experience is required to identify them because changes in the bone caused by cavitations are subtle and may actually look like normal bony anatomy. Osteonecrosis, a disease of the marrow spaces of bone, is serious and can sometimes destroy as much as 30 to 50 percent

---

* ZRT Laboratory.

† Quicksilver Scientific Testing Manual, http://www.quicksilverscientific.com/.

‡ Ronda Nelson, MPH, PHD, *Functional Blood Chemistry Manual* (Interpretation of CBC, CMP and Lipid Panels).

§ IAOMT, IABDM, Osteo-Cavitations, Seminars, conference notes, 2016.

of the bone before changes can be readily seen on an X-ray. Remember, X-rays give us a picture of hard tissue only.

Even MRIs do not provide a sure solution. MRI imaging scans work well for long bones, but the flat bones of the face are not imaged well with normal MRIs. A new ultrasound image technique called MRI-STIR imaging has shown remarkable accuracy in determining cavitation locations, and the newer, three-dimensional CBCT-3D scans are more effective in determining cavitation locations that are more difficult to see on a two-dimensional X-ray film. In both cases, surgical success is improved when using these imaging techniques.*

Another diagnostic technique is to have an oral surgeon anesthetize the suspect area. If the pain goes away after an anesthetic injection, then you can be reasonably certain there's a problem in the location that is generating the pain.

Although more than seventy risk factors have been identified as contributing to cavitation formation, in general, trauma and infection are the primary triggers for cavitation areas. The reason the issue is so acute with jaws and hip bones is that no other bones in the body come anywhere close to the amount of trauma and infection endured by the maxilla, mandible, and your hip bones.

Knowing that there are "general" causes, though, doesn't help you know how to manage cavitation problems if you have them. To be more specific, I've noted below a laundry list of potential causes, so that you can avoid them if possible or know what might be the trigger if you think you do have a problem.†

Causes of Cavitations

- **Trauma** from mild or severe direct blows to the jaw
- **Persistent tooth infections, chronically sensitive teeth** after dental restorations, or severe tooth infections
- **Surgical trauma** following extractions, especially wisdom teeth, endodontic surgery (such as root canals), and the like. If there is enough room for the eruption of your wisdom teeth and they are not periodontally involved, I would recommend leaving them in place.

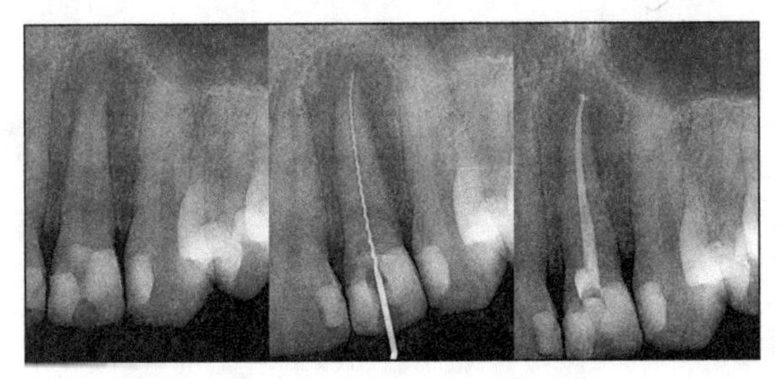

X-rays showing stages of endodontic treatment: before, during, and after. Credit: danielzgombic.

* Levy, *Hidden Epidemic.*

† George Meinig, DDS, FACD, *Root Canal Cover-up* (Price Pottenger Nutrition, 2008).

- **Thrombophilia and hypo-fibrinolysis.** These are genetic blood coagulation disorders that predispose some people to form blood clots, thereby preventing blood flow, which starves the bone of oxygen. The first condition, thrombophilia, increases the tendency to develop blood clots. The second condition, hypo-fibrinolysis, reduces the ability to destroy blood clots.
- **Failed root canals** or persistent infections following root canal therapy or dry sockets from wisdom tooth removal.
- **Antiphospholipid syndrome.** With this immune system disease, blood clots can develop within small arteries and veins. This condition creates a situation in which antibodies are manufactured and act against your body, often producing blood clots—and cavitations if the clots occur within the bone.
- **Extractions**—usually third molar extractions—but extraction of any tooth can create a problem, especially if dry sockets have occurred.

A serious concern is that cavitations may be completely painless. Chronic inflammation and swelling can occur in one or more of the tiny vessels producing the death of the vessels, then ischemia occurs, and ultimately bone death, before you even know you have a problem. As bad as that news is, there is some good news with regard to the treatability of cavitations. Here's a sampling of what can be done:

- **Surgery with protein rich plasma** (PRP). These are stem cells from your blood. The procedure involves removal of damaged tissue (surgical debridement) in the affected area and the introduction of PRP to facilitate the growth of new bone. We introduce ozonated gas and water during this step. This process removes the dead bone and bone marrow, kills all the pathogenic bugs, and creates a new environment for healing. (Note that all materials removed during the surgery should be biopsied.)
- **Hyperbaric therapy.** Similar to ozone therapy, this is a systemic treatment by which the patient is placed in a hyperbaric chamber, which raises the atmospheric pressure and drives oxygen into the cells of the body. (Used to reverse the bends in diving accidents.)
- **Anticoagulant therapy.** If you have a systemic clotting problem or other clotting risk factors, anticlotting medications can be administered.
- **Injection of homeopathic remedies.** This has become popular recently but is not a permanent solution because it does not correct the problem that dead bone has, which is having little to no blood supply. Adequate blood supply and increased NO is required for normal healing plus the removal of toxins.

- **Ozone therapy**—injections of ozone directly into the cavitation site (this tends to be highly effective). You can also drink ozone water or use a process called insufflation.
- **Natural antibiotic therapies.**

Even though I've said detection of cavitations can be difficult, it's not impossible.

Here is a list of symptoms and warning signs to keep in mind if you think you may be affected:

- Deep bone pain that is constant but varying in intensity.
- Sharp, shooting pain.
- Chronic maxillary sinusitis, including nasal congestion, pain, and drainage.
- A sour or bitter taste in the mouth, which can cause gagging and bad breath.
- A history of large fillings, followed by pain, then root canals, then removal of the tooth.
- Multiple root canals.
- Endodontic apicoectomy (removal of the root tip after a root canal).
- Tooth extraction, especially following a past dry socket or difficult extraction.
- Failed trigeminal neuralgia (facial pain) treatment. (This is because standard treatments do not address cavitations, so if the treatment fails to eliminate the facial pain, a cavitation may be the real culprit.)

The Urinary Filtrate

The material filtered through the kidneys is actually a blood product we call the urinary filtrate. The blood is filtered through the glomerulus (capillaries in the kidney), then is secreted into the collecting tubules of the kidney. When this filtrate is analyzed, it tells us what the body is getting rid of, what the body has in excess, and sometimes what the body doesn't have enough of.

The analogy here is like your checkbook ledger. When you want to see where your money has gone, you look at your checkbook ledger. When you want to see what your body has spent or the nutrients that have been metabolized, you look at the urinary metabolites.[*, †]

---

* A4M, 24th Annual World Congress on Anti-Aging Medicine, conference notes (Hollywood, FL, May 20–21, 2016).

† ZRT Laboratory.

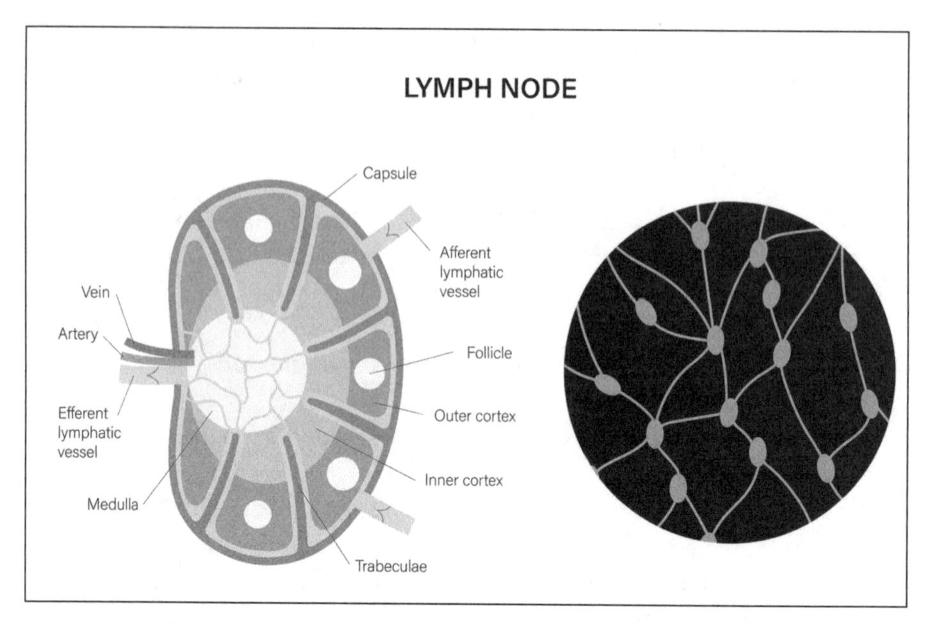

Anatomy of a lymph node and human lymphatic system infographic. Credit: Pikovit44.

If the kidneys are unable to get rid of spent wastes or toxins, fat cells must take over the storage process. Similar to the sugar storage we will talk about later on, these adipocytes (fat cells) store toxic waste to protect the body. And guess what happens in the process? You get fat, because your fat cells must dilute the toxins with water by swelling up. When the fat cells become overloaded, the excess waste is passed to the mesenchymal tissue. The problem here, though, is that this tissue is supposed to spend its time producing healthy lymphatic tissue rather than being in the toxin disposal business.

When all of these cellular systems and backup systems are full of toxins, then all of the junk spills out into organs themselves (the body's parenchymal tissue). This disrupts the proper functioning of the cells by reducing their ability for metabolism and self-repair. This creates a seriously poor cellular environment, and, as you can see, we're back to the problem of maintaining health at the cellular level.

A negative cell environment (recall the biological terrain) is a setup for the invasion of fungi, bacteria, pseudomonas, parasites, mycotoxins, viruses, and other noxious bugs. It also causes a cellular voltage drop, which inhibits the production of new cells. (This is a big problem.)

You must treat dysfunctional cellular metabolism to prevent over-acidity and over-alkalization of the blood. This is absolutely paramount to your overall health.

One very doable way to help your body accomplish this is to start fasting. When you fast, your body can dump whatever toxins are in your mesenchymal tissue into the blood. This is called CR or caloric restriction.

See the appendix for the benefits of CR.

The waste products you'll be getting rid of include:

- Xenobiotics
- Lactic acid
- Ketone bodies
- Toxins from an incomplete protein burn
- Toxins from an incomplete burn of fats (which causes lipid peroxidation that is highly damaging to your cells).

Fortunately, all of these toxins are dumped by the first morning void of your urine. That makes this the ideal time to test your urinary pH to find out if over-acidity is a problem. Another important measure is the specific gravity of urine because if the SG is too low, it could indicate the beginnings of kidney deficiency and a diminished ability to get rid of spent waste products and toxins from your body.*

The Truth About Root Canals

There is an ongoing battle regarding endodontic treatment for saving broken-down or infected teeth, but the seriously complicating factor is that, within a tooth, there are literally miles of lateral dentinal tubules, outside of the main canals, which remain unfilled after a root canal procedure.

These odontoblastic tubules (lateral canals) can harbor bacteria and their toxic end products, causing an infective process to stay active and smolder, undetected, for years. Infection can lay dormant within the tooth or rear its ugly head shortly after the procedure.

These bacterial endotoxins can enter your body's circulatory system and release cytokine modulators which can increase inflammation in every organ system in your body. Obviously, this is not good news.

For this reason, root canal therapy is a procedure that should very rarely, if ever, be performed under any circumstance, according to these highly credible sources:

- American Academy of Anti-Aging Medicine (A4M)
- International Academy of Oral Medicine & Toxicology (IAOMT)
- Holistic Dental Association (HDA)
- International Academy of Biological Dentistry & Medicine (IABDM)
- Institute for Functional Medicine (IFM)

* Quicksilver Scientific Protocols and Testing Manual, http://www.quicksilverscientific.com/.

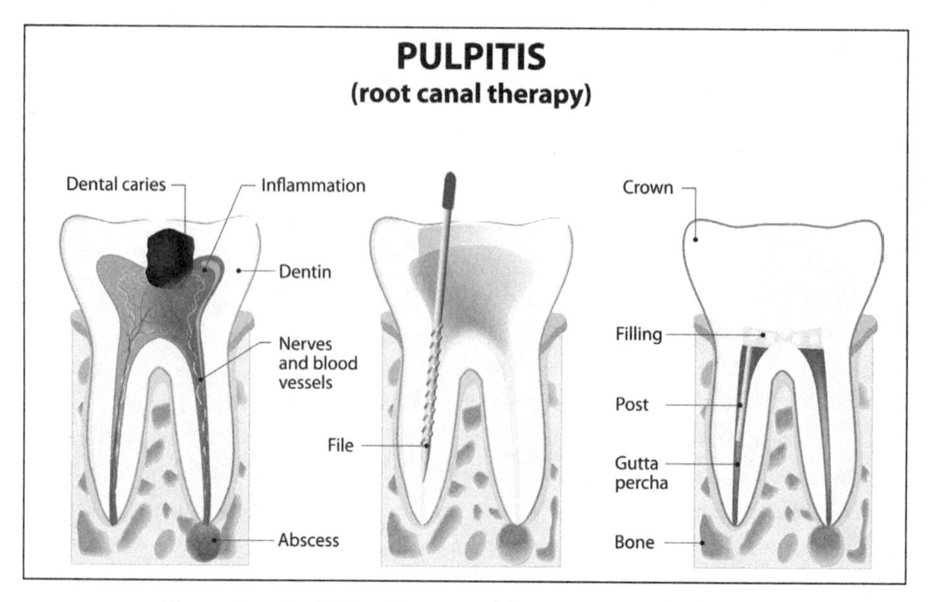

Illustration of pulpitis and root canal therapy process. Credit: ttsz.

Unfortunately, the American Dental Association (ADA) and the American Associations of Endodontics (AAE) disagree, and they, obviously, have major influence on what dentists do.

The whole issue boils down to this: Can a tooth be filled internally and remain uninfected years after the inside of the pulp canals have been filled? The biological dentistry camp (that includes me) says, no way. But the establishment dentistry camp says, absolutely yes. Let me explain in more detail why I think the biological dentistry camp has it right.

Your teeth have meridian channels through which each tooth has a connection to various organ systems. Any blockage of these meridians—such as caused by an infected root canal—causes problems in the associated organ. Breast cancer is one example of this connection gone wrong.[*, †, ‡]

Anterior teeth have simpler root canal systems while molars have very complicated root canal systems with multiple canals. This makes molar teeth more difficult to fill and much easier to fail in the end. In my clinical experience, I have seen endodontic failures as well as a few endodontic successes, but the problem is you can only fill the main canals and not all of the accessory canals which is where the bacteria and pathogenic bugs set up housekeeping.

Your teeth are like batteries, and when they become infected, the voltage and oxygenation in the infected tooth drops and as we've already discussed, healing

* Levy, *Hidden Epidemic.*

† Tennant, *Healing Is Voltage.*

‡ Laird Wellness, Root Canals and Breast Cancer, et al., https://rumble.com/v4vs7zb-root-canals-and-breast-cancer.html.

is impaired. Unfortunately, standard dentistry and medicine have yet to fully embrace this concept.

If you have had a root canal by an endodontist or a well-trained general dentist, follow up with an X-ray or a CBCT scan to evaluate the end of the root and to check for infection. Then discuss the findings with a biological dentistry office.

For an educational explanation on root canals, review the documentary, *Root Cause.*[*] If you haven't had a root canal but think you have a tooth that is a candidate for one, you might do well with the procedure if your immune system is not compromised—especially if your practitioner will use ozone therapy as part of the procedure. The fact is, if you want to save your tooth or absolutely must save it, the only option is root canal therapy.

You just need to go into the procedure knowing the downside and doing the best you can to ensure the best possible results (I rarely recommend root canals, for instance, unless ozone is used at the same time). If you elect to have an RCT performed, my advice is to seek the service of an endodontic specialist.

If your situation is already a problem—i.e., your present root canal is infected—you need to have it removed properly, by a biological dentistry specialist who will remove the periodontal ligament. Then consider which of the three alternatives you will pursue:

1. Implant placement and crown, preferably ceramic implants
2. All porcelain bridge construction
3. Flexible removable partial denture (these are made from nylon-based material and look very aesthetic with no metals or BPA plastics)

Ultimately, the decision on what to do is yours. Just don't be coerced into taking a course of action you aren't convinced is right for you.

Biofilm, Bacteria, Nutritional Deficiencies, and Dental Decay

Contrary to what you may have been told, dentistry has been trying to figure out, for decades, exactly what causes dental caries, better known as tooth decay. It stands as one of the top health problems globally. We do know that, along with gingivitis and periodontal disease, caries are related to bacterial biofilm, pH, and the DFTS.[†]

To illustrate how this works: A good example of a well-organized bacterial biomass is the underside of a boat or barge that has been sitting in the water for many months. The hull is covered with rust, barnacles, oxidized slime, mold, and nasty parasitic microbes. This "coating" on the boat is like the biofilm on your

---

* *The Root Cause*, https://tubitv.com/movies/507721/root-cause.

† ADA, Journal of the American Dental Association, Caries Risk Assessment and Management, The Harvard Study (2001); https://www.ada.org/resources/ada-library/oral-health-topics/caries-risk-assessment-and-management.

teeth. Biofilm is a serious coconspirator in the causation of dental caries. Better known as plaque, this slimy, sticky layer of film adheres to the teeth and gums and is hard to penetrate with alkalinizing agents (like toothpaste). Another culprit in dental caries is the acidification of saliva. When the pH of saliva becomes too acidic, below 5.5, it favors the growth of destructive bacteria which attack the enamel, gingival surfaces (the gums), and bone.

Dental infections (i.e., decay) are acidic and they carry a positive (+) electrical charge. Minerals also carry a positive charge and therefore are blocked because the infection repels the entry of the minerals into the areas of the tooth that are infected (positive charges repel other positive charges). This process is known as demineralization, and just like it sounds, it removes necessary minerals from your teeth. On the other hand, an alkaline (i.e., healing) environment carries a negative charge and will therefore accept minerals, with a positive charge into the teeth and bone. This is called remineralization and is why ozone therapy is so effective.*

These are the keys to healthy mineralization of the teeth:

1. Mineral ratios must be in the correct balance to counteract enamel demineralization of your teeth and bones. This also prevents osteoporosis in other bones in the body.
2. Maintain developmental nutritional substrates. Weston A. Price, DDS, proved years ago that populations devoid of nutrient substrates had lots of dental crowding and decay issues.†
3. Keep the dentinal fluid transport system operating efficiently by avoiding refined sugars. Sugar is a food source for destructive bacteria and fungus in your mouth, upper respiratory tract, throat, and sinus areas, and it promotes candida growth. Pearl Nature's Toothpaste® is a mineralizing toothpaste and it is anti-biofilm.‡
4. Correct crowded, deficient arch forms and crooked teeth. A crowded arch form, either upper or lower, contributes to poor oral healthcare, mouth breathing, deep overbites, poor TMJ positioning, OSA, and the retention of bacteria in the hard-to-clean areas of your mouth.
5. Daily oral healthcare. If the biomass is not removed every day, acid contained in the biofilm establishes itself on the tooth and gum surfaces and begins to organize in a way that can cause infection.
6. Correct mouth breathing by widening the dental arches.

---

* Roggenkamp, *Dentinal Fluid Transport.*

† Weston A. Price, DDS, *Nutrition and Physical Degeneration, 1939* (Price-Pottenger Nutrition Foundation Publishing, 2008).

‡ http://www.PearlOralHealth.com.

So, these are the many aspects of the "window to your health" that occur inside your mouth, and as I've said, standard dental procedures generally do not address the real issues involved. But there are many ways to take good care of your overall health, including widening of constricted dental arches early in development, which I'll explain in the second half of chapter 4.

CHAPTER 4

What Is Antiaging Medicine and Dentistry?

Antiaging medicine is a clinical, medical specialty and field of scientific research aimed at the early detection, prevention, treatment, and reversal of age-related decline. It is well documented by peer-reviewed medical and scientific journals and employs evidence-based methodologies to conduct patient assessments. Chronological age is not the only—or even the primary—determinant of a person's biological age. Your biological age is determined by the performance of your cellular metabolism. That's why antiaging medicine focuses on identifying the cellular markers that can determine how old you really are on the inside.

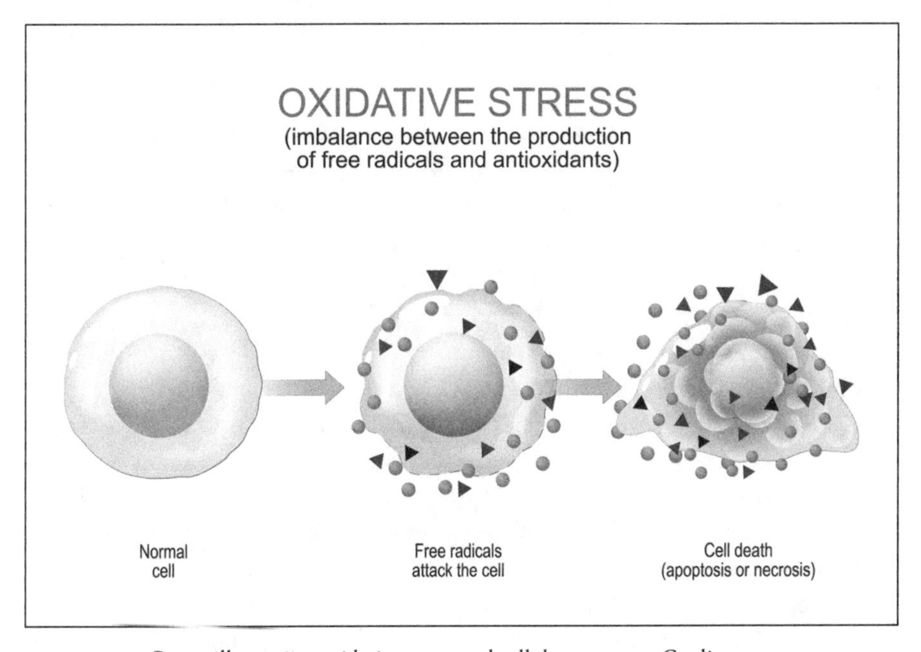

Poster illustrating oxidative stress and cellular response. Credit: ttsz.

The Importance of Free Radical Oxidation

Free radical oxidative stress occurs in all cells and produces the free radical exhaust of cellular energy production. That means, as your cells burn oxygen to produce energy, they give off toxic biological waste products in the form of free radicals.

Technically speaking, free radicals are singlet, unbound elements of oxygen that have an electron missing from their chemical makeup. This makes them unstable and potentially damaging because an unstable element will "look for" a means to stabilize itself and will bind to another electron—which should be used for other purposes—if need be. The unchecked presence of free radicals is a significant factor in the aging process.

Aging is further complicated by the body's fluctuating hormonal levels. Through time, healthful hormonal levels tend to decrease, while two harmful hormones, insulin and cortisol, increase. This is why a protocol known as bioidentical hormone replacement therapy (BIHRT) is one of the foundations of antiaging medicine for both men and women. BIHRT is one of the best ways of controlling silent inflammation, the fundamental result of hormonal imbalance, free radicals, and other internal health-damaging conditions. Dinosaur docs who claim that synthetic hormones as well as BIHRT produce cancer are just flat-out wrong. If your doctor tells you BIHRT is not the way to go, you need a new physician. While BIHRT is often not covered by traditional medical insurance, ask yourself whether you want to use your insurance or if you want to get well.

The Optimal Health Continuum

As we've already discussed, optimal health starts at the cellular level. Our focus on maintaining cellular-level health is as important in the early years of your life (from birth to thirty years of age)—perhaps even more than—it is in later years. Yet, chronic disease, on which roughly 50 percent of the US healthcare dollar is spent, generally develops later because of poor early conditions and has become the main focus of contemporary symptom-based medical practices. But at this juncture, the best the medical system can offer is a way to play catch-up—and usually with treatments that still do not address the core problem, cellular metabolism. This end-stage focus of the health continuum represents a state of extreme illness or premature death of cells—called apoptosis—whereas the beginning of the health continuum represents a state of greater optimal health.

Traditional medicine has almost exclusively focused on the illness side while health promotion focuses on the optimal health side of the continuum.

In the early stages of life, our God-given DNA causes us to grow. It's called the anabolic phase. After age thirty or forty, we enter the catabolic stage in which things begin to slow down.

Oddly enough, the lack of focus on the cellular level of health is not because cell health is a mystery. In truth, we know a great deal about cellular integrity.

Cellular metabolic markers show us what is happening inside the cells, and if we pay attention and grasp the appropriate ways to handle what we see, enzymes, hormones, minerals, and other benchmarks tell us exactly what we need to know to restore our health. The trouble is that symptom-based medicine and dentistry practitioners are not trained to measure metabolic function. And as we said before, neither are hospitals.

To give you a quick example: Gut flora in the digestive system is a mixture of good bacteria that determines how well you absorb nutrients, maintain immunities, and eliminate waste, among other things. The proper balance in the gut can be established through certain dietary and supplemental protocols that lead to a healthy digestive system.[*]

This is foundational to good health because the processes that lead to disease begin in the gut, and your gut begins in your mouth.

Age Rejuvenation: A Legacy of Good Health

More than two thousand years ago, the famous Greek physician and scientist Hippocrates said, "Let your food be your medicine and your medicine be your food." He understood that what we take into our bodies has a drastic effect on our health. Yet this is an idea that has been lost through the ages.

This also includes the loss of ancient Hebrew dietary laws found in the Holy Bible (He put them there for a reason). If you read the book *Kosher* by Todd Bennett,[†] I guarantee you will stop eating "unclean" foods.[‡] Other than a few peripheral (and often incorrect) recommendations, modern presciption-pad medicine docs generally ignore the central truth of Hippocrates's teaching. Why? Can you say "modern agribusiness?" They think that Ensure is really food, amazing! To them nutrition is just for moms whom are out on a limb wasting way too much time on the internet worrying about their children. Well, I'm here to tell you these moms are dead on the money and that collectively they know more about natural health than most practitioners do. I see it in my busy practice, and I learn a lot from them every day.

Today, however, we have an expensive, ineffective, arrogant bureaucratically driven approach to medicine that has taken the place of personal responsibility for one's health. As a result, no one even knows what the direct cost of healthcare is to our society, let alone the indirect cost in lost health, inability to work, and premature death. Functional dentistry and integrative medicine can vastly improve the quality of life, especially as we age.

In my Forty-Eight Medical and Dental Myopic Myths I've outlined, by implication, how far down the wrong path we have been led and at the end of

---

* Dr. Josh Axe, Eat Dirt! (HarperCollins Publishers, 2016).

† Todd D. Bennett, *Kosher*. Walk in the Light Series (Shema Yisrael Publications, 2005).

‡ Holy Bible, Lev 20: 25, 26 (KJV).

this chapter I counter those myths with Thirty-Two Ways to Reverse the Aging Process. Which is to say that we can recapture the vision for our health set before us twenty centuries ago. And now, we can do better than ever because we do know so much more about how our bodies operate. Hopefully, this book is already raising your awareness of the need to address your particular health issues.

Today, more than ever, we know that true health is due to great nutrition, proper enzyme signaling, gut function, and proper detoxification, and less a result of overall genetics. Think of food as information for your on-and-off cytoplasmic genetic transcription switches that upregulate and downregulate your body chemistry. This is termed epigenetics and nutrigenomics and has a lot to do with how healthy or unhealthy you become.

The answer to good health is good food, but there's no place given in our modern medical paradigm for the proper use of food as "medicine." God created the puzzle and its solutions, yet we have virtually ignored the built-in answers to health problems.

Even though good nutritional medicine is not widely practiced commercially, the good news is that there are a growing number of forward-thinking, nutritionally astute doctors who have the same passion I do for natural health solutions. And patients like you are the other real key component of making this new approach viable. Especially you awesome "Crunchy Moms."

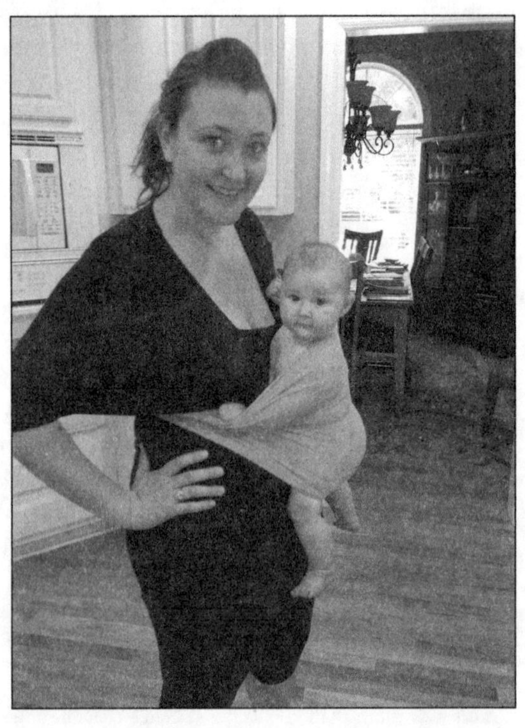

Angela and Evelyn Mishler. Credit: Jan Lokensgard

(My daughter and granddaughter are among them) I love you gals! Why? Because, unlike those following the path of traditional medicine, you play an active role in your and your family's good health. To make it work for you, you need three things: knowledge, personal responsibility, and commitment.

This book—and the larger program I mentioned earlier—will benefit anyone who wants to learn the very latest in natural healthcare. In the traditional, standard modern approach, we confuse detection with disease prevention, but early detection is not prevention. The approach I'm talking about is prevention, so that there's nothing to detect. That is a tall order, but in the end, I do believe it is achievable.

Prevention and Aging

Ultimately, as we prevent disease, we reduce the effects of aging. So, I'll conclude this chapter by outlining antiaging practices to guide you on the journey to a youthful new you. You may already be doing some of these things I've noted here, but the checklist will give you a way to see where you are on the road to true health.

Thirty-Two Ways to Reverse the Aging Process

1. Alkalinity and acidity balance coordinated with inflammation and obesity control (NF-k-Beta)
2. Energy production through cellular ATP and proper oxygen metabolism
3. Autoimmune control by balancing of secretory Ig-A and the microbiome
4. Cellular hydration through use of bio-energized water. This is noteworthy because our bodies are 70 percent water, and our brain bioplasm is 85 percent water. Getting healthy water into our bodies is important.
5. Blood sugar control and controlling the metabolic syndrome
6. Maintaining proper blood viscosity—Zeta-Spin Potential (ZSP), Nattokinase, and garlic
7. Bone porosity and electromagnetic therapy (EMT); balancing EMF and increasing silica with Pearl Silica Drops®
8. Maintaining cellular membrane integrity and ion channels and balancing the redox potential by increasing voltage via earthing (e.g., walking barefoot on grass, sand, or dirt)
9. Proper cell-receptor site sensitivity—receptor signaling, especially insulin receptors

(Continued on next page)

10. Managing chelation, zeolites, and heavy metal toxicity and reducing dental infections
11. Detoxification and liver cleansing (cleaning your oil filter, including your kidneys and gall bladder)
12. Dietary endocrinology, because you are what you eat and absorb (proper nutrient absorption is critical)
13. DNA protection, via methylation and MTHF Reductase testing and SNPs testing (fifty-six gene SNPs)
14. Enzyme balance for proper digestion and metabolism
15. Free radical oxidative stress (FROS) control
16. Hormonal balance, because hormones are the symphony conductor for the whole body
17. Inflammatory control and control of NF-k-Beta protein for immune function
18. Maintaining proper iodine levels as well as salt and mineral levels, including selenium and PQQ support 20mg per day
19. Keeping LGS, stomach pH, probiotics, and the microbiome at optimal levels
20. Muscle mass, BIA, BMI, VPP, vibrational power plate usage, and increasing nitric oxide[*]
21. Balancing the NEI axis—the neuro-, endocrine, and immune axis
22. Limit the loss of brain voltage by neurogenesis to optimize neurotransmitter balance, nootropics, and brain-derived neurogenic factor (BDNF), which helps with a process called neuroplasticity (new nerve growth)
23. Nutrigenomics, because what you eat affects your gene transcription switches
24. O_2 use and heart rate variability (HRV)
25. Controlling stress through the parasympathetic and sympathetic nervous systems, implementing the Wim Hof breathing techniques[†] or Buteyko breathing method[‡]
26. Maintaining periodontal health with ozone and saturated salt solution (ozone therapies)

---

* Scott Laird, ND and Jodi Laird; Laird Wellness; Nitric Oxide: The Miracle Molecule, https://rumble.com/v31sisg-nitric-oxide-the-miracle-molecule.html.

† Wim Hof, *The Wim Hof Method: Activate Your Full Human Potential* (Sounds True, June 28, 2022).

‡ Ralph Skuban, PhD; *The Buteyko Method: How to Improve Your Breathing for Better Health and Performance in All Areas of Life* (Based on 1960s research by Ukrainian physician Dr. Konstantin Buteyko, 1923–2003) (Skuban Academy; 1st edition (February 14, 2024).

27. Keeping phytonutrient and glycoprotein integrity intact with eight essential nutrients, the glyco-phospholipids, and by improving your biological terrain
28. Helping the energy cycle through mitochondrial support with PQQ and CR
29. Sirtuin gene suppression by trans-resveratrol and EGCG, found in green tea extract
30. Maintaining healthful sleep by eliminating obstructive sleep apnea (OSA) and by finding insomnia solutions
31. Stress and HPA control for adrenal support and fatigue management
32. Using vitamin D3 (it's an amazing hormone, not just a vitamin), get your levels to 80 to 100 ng/ml, use the ZRT test or the Dutch test

There are modules that detail all of these methodologies. The more of these you can do, the better off you'll be, and I'll explain more about what you can do as we go.

FUNCTIONAL JAW ORTHOPEDIC ORTHODONTICS

Optimizing oxygen levels is vital for overall health, including long-term anti-aging benefits. To achieve this, reducing mouth breathing and promoting nasal breathing is key. Proper jaw alignment facilitates better nasal airflow, reducing reliance on mouth breathing and improving oxygen intake.

WHAT IS CRANIOFACIAL ORTHOPEDICS?

One of the most important topics in dentistry today is oral-facial myology and oral-facial growth. I say this because there are so many complications that can and do occur later in life if the face is not fully formed or grows improperly in a child's developmental years.

Facial orthopedics has the potential to improve functional conditions, promote more favorable jaw positioning, guide the development of dentition, and improve the position of misaligned teeth. This allows for more favorable placement of:

- TMJs
- The nose
- The teeth
- The chin
- The lower face
- The sinuses
- The dental arches

To repeat: Growth and great health are dependent on oxygen consumption and efficient metabolism, which is dependent on proper facial growth and jaw size, which can be corrected by craniofacial orthopedic-orthodontics early in life. The window for best facial development is from birth through twelve years of age.

So, to you awesome moms out there: If your baby won't or can't latch, if his or her teeth come in crowded or they have deep bites and tongue-ties, bring them to a practitioner who understands myo-facial orthodontic development.

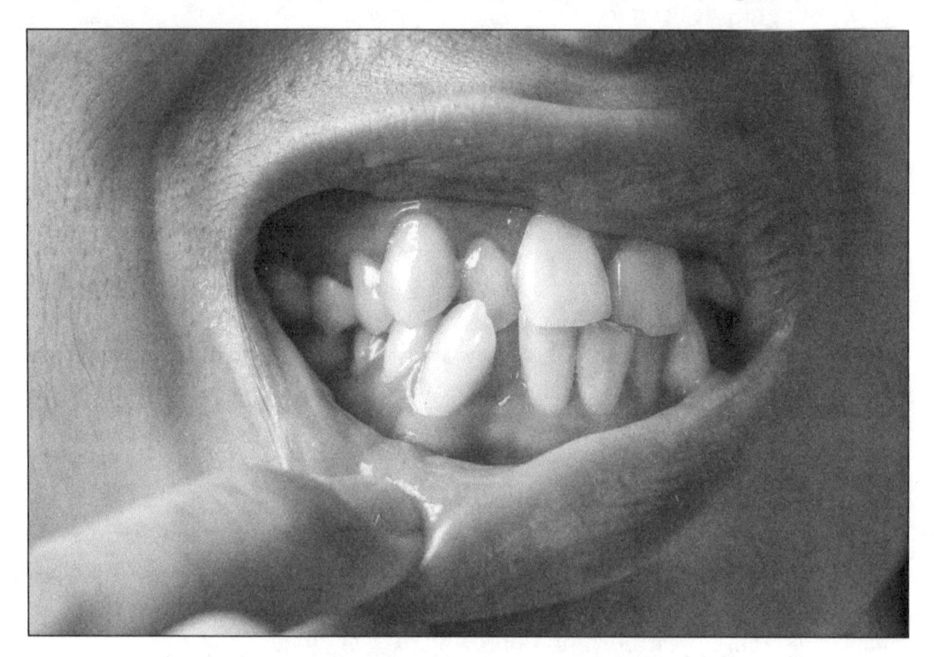

Close-up of crowded teeth. Credit: Zay Nyi Nyi.

The Good Lord designed us to be nose breathers. If the jaws are too narrow, and the tongue can't reach the palate due to a tongue-tie, the maxilla (upper jaw) won't develop to its proper size, and the mandible (lower jaw) will drop to the back of the throat, thereby causing a pharyngeal airway obstruction and decreased oxygen consumption, plus fatigue. This is just the beginning of a long list of potential problems.*

Next, during the day, the tongue begins to protrude through the upper and lower teeth, contributing to potential speech issues, a narrower and shorter lower face height and extremely crowded teeth. At night, the tongue again flops back into the throat, contributing to snoring, obstructed sleep apnea, and mouth breathing, which continues the lack of oxygen consumption, fatigue, and

* IAO (International Association of Orthodontics) Practitioner Advancement Course, conference notes, (http://www.iaortho.org/).

a decrease in overall metabolism which directly lowers ATP production in the Krebs cycle!

It gets worse. The sinuses do not develop because of improper air flow and critical air exchange that doesn't cool off the sinuses and impinges on the pineal gland and the pituitary gland, which are absolutely essential for whole-body growth and development. Get the picture? So, here's the deal. Breast feed your baby. It helps them to develop their jaws, become nose breathers, and grow to their God-given potential.

Functional Orthodontics or Early Interceptive Orthodontics

Today, orthodontists, pediatric dentists and general dentists are discussing and treating orthopedic problems in the mixed dentition (early facial development) phase, because e*arly treatment is superior treatment.* Some orthodontic practitioners gear their practices to treatment in the permanent dentition only. This completely misses a window of opportunity to capitalize on facial growth plates.

We believe that capitalizing on facial growth is SUPERIOR TREATMENT!

Clearly, any orthopedic problem, such as a constricted (narrow) upper arch, a retrognathic mandible (displaced chin), or a deep overbite is much easier to treat in the mixed dentition. When treatment is instituted early, 80 percent of the malocclusions (bad bites) can be treated with orthopedic expansion appliances and the remaining 20 percent solved with the straight wire appliance (fixed braces).

This two-phase treatment approach ensures that in excess of 95 percent of our mixed dentition cases can be treated without extraction and nonsurgically.

What are Some of the Functional Orthopedic Issues?

1. Dental cross-bites
2. Underdeveloped arches (upper and lower jaws)
3. Crowded teeth and tongue-ties
4. Airway constriction
5. Large tonsils and mouth breathing
6. TMJ Problems
7. Deep bites or recessive bites

These problems should be corrected earlier rather than later. When we correct out these growth issues through orthopedic expansion you can sleep, breathe, and talk better. The self-esteem factor will also improve with this procedure. The end results that we see in our clinic are nothing short of fantastic. I recommend slow palatal expansion as opposed to rapid palatal expansion.

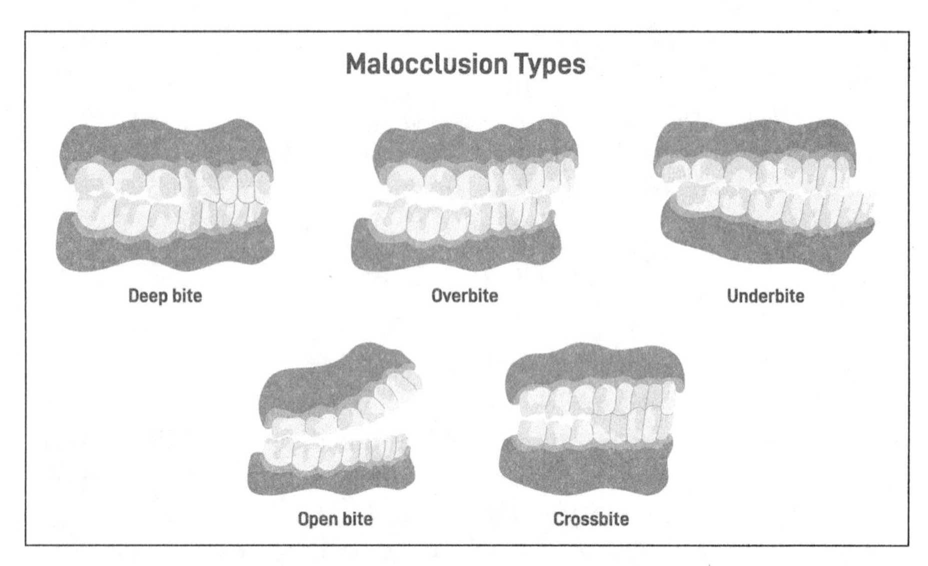

Malocclusion types. Credit: Guzaliia Filimonova.

Eight Keys to Facial Beauty and TMJ Health

There are many advantages of using functional orthodontics for your children. Below is a summary of the advantages:

Functional Jaw Orthopedics (FJOs)

1. Proper maxillary arch width and arch form
2. Proper maxillary anterior-posterior position (overbite and overjet)
3. Proper maxillary A-P position in relation to properly located maxilla (upper jaw)
4. Proper vertical dimension (lower face height)
5. Mandibular symmetry (front views) facial profile
6. Proper uprighting of lower posterior teeth and proper lower arch form (upper buccal quadrants)
7. Proper condylar position
8. Level maxillary occlusal plane

Functional Jaw Orthopedics Solves:

1. Functional habits (muscles)
2. Skeletal problems (bone)
3. Dental problems (teeth)
4. TMJ problems (joints)
5. Airway problems (breathing)

Advantages of Functional Jaw Orthopedics (FJOs)

1. Less dental decay than with fixed appliances (braces)
2. Can start in mixed dentition stage (early intervention)

3. Addresses both orthopedic and orthodontic problems of malocclusion
4. Puts the bones and the teeth in the right place while readapting the musculature
   a. The theory is that improper muscle functioning does not allow proper growth and alignment of the jaws, thus causing orthopedic misalignment of apical bases and dental crowding. By changing the function of those muscles and the forces they impact on the teeth and the basal bone, you change the shape of the bones back to their normal inter-arch alignment and size. A size large enough to accommodate all of the naturally existing teeth.
   b. FJOs corrects the malposed teeth and malposed bone and readapts the musculature. This technique is the most facially oriented orthodontic technique.
5. Beautiful, broad smile
6. Excellent functional occlusion
7. Full face with beautiful jawlines and lateral profile
8. Sound, healthy TMJs
9. Nonsurgical; without extraction (less time in braces)
10. Strong chin and facial profile because you are rounding out the facial architecture
11. Retaining twenty-eight teeth instead of twenty-four
12. Growth of the mandible occurs in the condylar head and neck, based on computerized serial radiographic analysis and scientific studies

To summarize, using functioning orthodontics does not perpetuate "natural mistakes" of the original malocclusion, resulting in proper arch form and thereby increasing oxygen flow.

ORTHODONTICS: THREE-PHASE TREATMENT

In our practice we use a three-phase treatment approach

1. Phase 1 Orthopedics (Bone development)
   - developing the upper and lower arch form to fit the teeth

2. Phase 2 Orthodontics (Brackets or aligners)
   - lining up your teeth like railroad cars on a train track

3. Phase 3 Retention (The holding phase)
   - holding your teeth in their new position

Today, capitalizing on the growth plates, much like the tectonic plates in the earth's crust, gives us a substantial advantage in changing facial dynamics.

Today, we are treating orthopedic problems in the mixed dentition, early in life.

Early treatment is superior treatment. Here's why:

Two leading orthodontic researchers, Dr. Donald Woodside (Toronto, Ontario) and Dr. James McNamara* (Ann Arbor, Michigan), worked extensively with adolescent monkeys and functional jaw repositioning appliances and reported that condylar changes only occurred when the monkeys were actively growing. The research clearly demonstrates that today's orthopedic clinicians will obtain the ultimate response while the patient is actively growing. This is when the growth plates are active and the reason why earlier treatment is superior treatment.

Clearly, any orthopedic problem such as a constricted maxillary arch, a retrognathic mandible, or a deep overbite is much easier to treat in the mixed dentition phase. When treatment is instituted early, 80 percent of the malocclusions can be treated with orthopedic appliances and the remaining 20 percent solved with the straight wire appliance (fixed braces) or clear-correct, orthodontic trays.

This three-phase treatment approach ensures that in excess of 95 percent of our mixed dentition cases can be treated without extraction and nonsurgically. The third phase is the retention phase.

The bottom line is that if we want the best treatment for our younger patients, we must treat orthopedic problems such as transverse, sagittal, vertical, or functional problems in the mixed dentition stage, prior to the eruption of the permanent teeth.

The end result is that the newly widened dentition, which is done slowly over time, is much more stable and less likely to relapse.[†, ‡, §]

Orthodontic Appliances

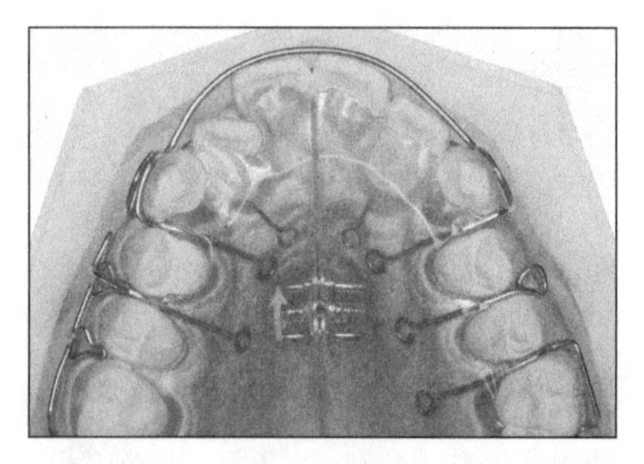

Upper orthopedic appliance. Credit: Hightower_NRW.

---

* James A. McNamara, DDS, MS, PhD, and Donald G. Woodside, DDS, researchers, https://dent.umich.edu/directory/mcnamara, https://pocket dentistry.com/donald-garth-woodside-a-leader-for-orthodontic-research-and-education-in-canada/.

† AAFO (An Advanced Field of Orthodontics) Seminar Training notes, http://www.aafo.org/.

‡ IAO, Practitioner Advancement Course, conference lecture notes, http://www.iaortho.org/.

§ IAOMT, conference lecture notes, 2018.

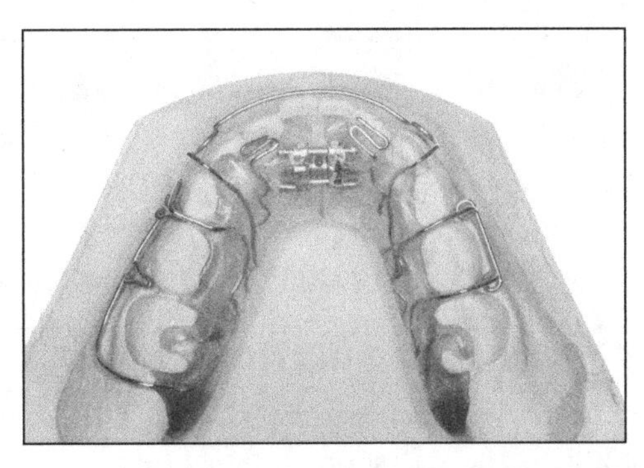

Lower orthopedic appliance. Credit: Hightower_NRW.

CRANIOSACRAL THERAPY

Andrew Taylor Still, MD, was a pioneering doctor. Unsatisfied with the medicine that he practiced, he developed the concept and the importance of the movement of the spine. He established osteopathic medicine in 1874. William G. Sutherland, DO, developed cranial osteopathy. He developed the concept of the respiratory mechanism of the nervous system. In traditional Western medicine it is believed that the cranial bones fuse in childhood. Since 1874, osteopathic doctors, on the other hand, have been taught that the cranial bones move in a rhythmic pattern. There is a pump within the skull that runs down the spine called the craniosacral pump. Each time this pump is activated, it sends a surge of electrons throughout the body.*

Here's the deal:

1. The central nervous system, comprised of the brain and the spinal cord, has an inner, inherent rhythmic motion.
2. The cerebrospinal fluid (CSF) fluctuates, or moves back and forth in a relatively closed container called the central nervous system (CNS).
3. There are twenty-six bones in the head. All of them have a slight rhythmic motion along with the CNS, CSF, membranes, and sacrum. These bones all fit together like a jigsaw puzzle and influence each other. They are like tectonic plates.
4. Since the dura mater is attached to the base of the skull and the sacrum or tailbone, the motion of the cranial mechanism is transmitted to the sacrum. The cranium and the sacrum work together as one unit.

What this all means is that the cranial bones of the head move with the pulse of the nervous system. The sphenoid bone is the center of the system. As the sphenoid bone and the sacrum move, the cerebrospinal fluid circulates through the brain and the spinal cord.

* Tennant, et al., 166–70.

The sphenoid bone is the keystone for the skull. The position of the sphenoid bone dictates the center of gravity of the skull. When it shifts, it causes the other cranial bones to shift as well, and it moves the center of gravity of the skull. This causes the brain to send a signal to the neck, particularly the upper cervical vertebra, to move to get under the center of gravity of the skull so it won't fall over. This dictate from the brain changes the anatomical alignment of the whole body.*

HOW DO WE MOVE TEETH ORTHODONTICALLY?

Today, there are three primary routes that we use, but it all boils down to what we are trying to accomplish. The orthodontic routes are:

1. **Functional appliances** for upper and lower jaw widening and tooth uprighting and correcting vertical problems also called deep bites.
2. **Orthodontic brackets** (braces) with a series of wires to align your bite.
3. **CAD-CAM clear aligners** (these are clear trays that replace bracket and wire therapy).

We often use a combination of all three methods, depending on your stage of facial development. You see, it's not just about having straight teeth; it's all about having a great smile, a wide arch to create proper mouth breathing, proper TMJ positioning, and the correct bite.

The antiquated method of orthodontics, where we pulled four perfectly good premolars and four wisdom teeth is, in my opinion, a thing of the past. If the ultimate goal is to line up your teeth and you do not need any dental arch development, then aligners or brackets will work very well.

If you have crowded arches or TMJ issues, then it is much more likely we will use the functional appliance route first, then finish the bite with brackets or aligner therapy. Most often, we use combinations of the aforementioned three techniques.

* Tennant, et al., 165–170.

PART TWO

Principles of Anti-Aging and Functional Medicine

CHAPTER 5

Optimum Oral Health for Life

There seems to be a predisposition among both medical practitioners and patients alike that all the best medical techniques are new. In fact, most people would probably assume that virtually all of the most effective treatments for disease and injury have been developed in the last one hundred years. While it's true that medical science has made astounding leaps forward in the past century (especially, as I pointed out earlier, in the realm of trauma medicine), the fact is that many extremely effective and often more healthful treatments have simply been forgotten in the race to adopt new (and in many cases, more lucrative) ways of handling disease. So, as we discuss optimal oral health, it's important that you set aside any new-is-better-than-old preconceptions you may have.

Ozone: An (Oxygen) Blast from the Past

In 1857, *The Lancet*, a British medical journal, published a series of articles extolling the successful use of medical oxygen. The remarkable findings of these nineteenth-century doctors were put to use in Germany in the 1950s for the treatment of cancer. So, what were these practitioners doing? They were using what would now be called bio-oxidative therapy, the application of a special form of oxygen called ozone to the treatment of disease and infection.*

You've probably heard of the ozone layer in the upper atmosphere that is there to do beneficial things for life on earth, and for medical purposes, we're talking about the same substance. Ozone is a molecule that consists of three atoms of oxygen (O_3), as opposed to the usual two-atom molecule (O_2) that we normally breathe. The extra atom of oxygen gives this molecule some remarkably beneficial properties.

Cancer and other diseases simply cannot survive or thrive in an oxygen-rich environment. A highly oxygenated body is essentially immune to disease and can actually destroy already-existing disease. We can use ozone to create just such an environment in the body—in your biological terrain. It thereby creates

* Sears, *Confidential Cures Newsletter.*

conditions conducive to healing for dental infections as well as for creating a whole-body ecology which favors health over disease.

The essential reason ozone works so well is that bugs, bacteria, viruses, fungi, parasites, and spirochetes cannot survive in a high-oxygen environment. They need low, or no, oxygen levels to thrive. Infections in your teeth, periodontal tissue, gums, failed root canals, bone, and elsewhere in your body flourish because those areas are mostly devoid of oxygen. These low-oxygen sites attract anaerobic bacteria that cause infection. These bacteria, though, cannot handle an oxidative burst, so when you introduce O_3 into the site, it kills all of the pathogenic bugs.

Infections are areas that have an acidic or positive (+) charge, thereby repelling other positively charged ions, like minerals. This is why infected areas continue to demineralize. In this state, the minerals cannot flow into the infected area because of the charge. However, when the biological terrain is changed in the infected site to an alkaline, negatively charged, oxygen-containing environment, not only do the bugs die but the remineralization process begins. And it's the negative O_3 charge that kills the bad bacteria.*

Since bugs have no antioxidants in their cellular membranes, the ozone creates peroxide molecules which cause the bug membranes to burst and die. The application of oxygen with an additional oxygen atom (O_3) makes the molecule highly reactive, thereby causing the creation of peroxide-oxygen molecules called reactive oxygen species (ROS). A normal cell can handle this peroxide bombardment (to a point) because normal cells contain antioxidants, but bacteria and the like do not.†

Another benefit of ozone is its ability to increase the microvasculature in the affected area by increasing nitric oxide. This brings more blood flow into the area via the growth and stimulation of new vasculature (blood vessels) called capillaries. It is essentially enhancing the infrastructure of your body thereby boosting your oxygen metabolism and an enzyme called ENOS, which stimulates production of NO.

The injections of ozone gas are usually quite painless and take just a few minutes to deliver. Depending on the severity of the infection being treated, they need to be repeated every seven to ten days. My dental practice now uses ozone water in our periodontal program and for the remineralization of teeth even in very young children. We also use ozone gel.

Here's how the ozone treatment works. As we flow O_3 gas and water over the dentinal tubules in the cavity preparation, we sterilize the tubules and begin the healing process in the area being treated. The ozone destroys the bacteria involved in the decay and infective process, as it cleans and disinfects the area.

---

* Roggenkamp.

† Frank Shallenberger, MD, HMD, *Bursting with Energy* (Basic Health Publications, Inc., 2022).

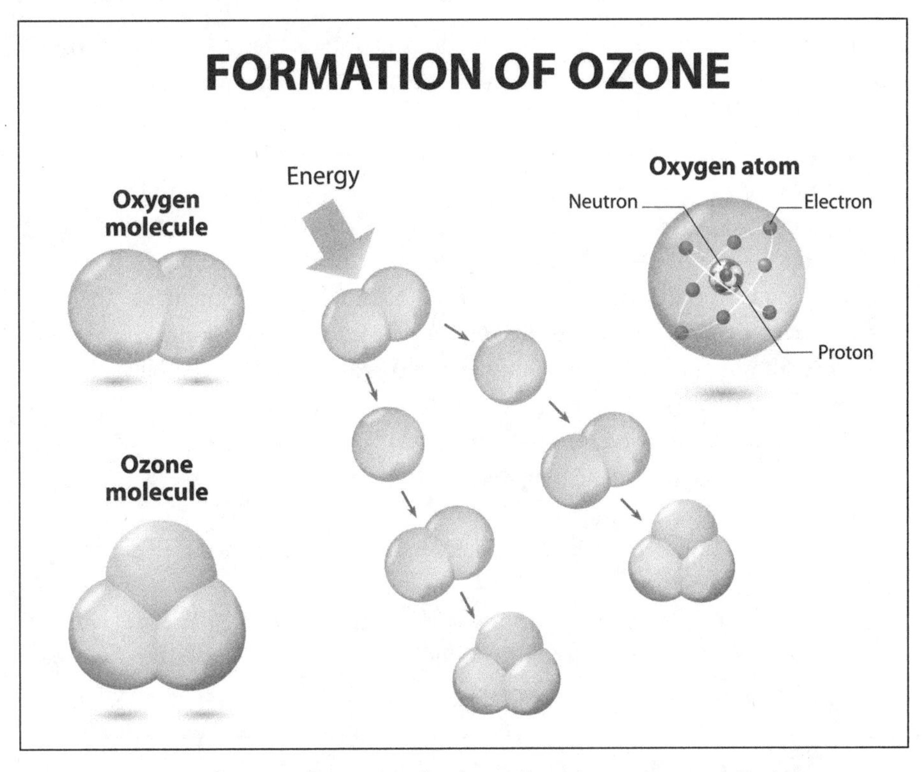

Illustration of ozone and oxygen molecules in photochemical process. Credit: ttsz.

We use ozone in our office to arrest tooth decay, periodontal disease, TMJD, and dystonia issues, oral surgery, infected cavitations, and root canals. To prepare for treatment, we create ozone water and ozone gas from medical-grade oxygen with a DOU-120 ozone machine. We also use tri-ozonated olive oil in ozone applications. In some cases, we can prepare ozone water that can be administered by the patient at home. We also use ozone to disinfect and to inject into areas with osteo-cavitations.*

Zeolites: What Are They, and How Do They Function?

Zeolites are heavy metal chelators, which means they are chemical compounds good at combining with other compounds. This offers a variety of benefits to the body. And speaking of "old" things that are good for modern medicine, zeolites are naturally occurring minerals formed from the remnants of ancient volcanic activity by the pressure and cooling of volcanic rock.

The advantage they offer derives from their small size and negative charge which enables zeolites to trap toxic metals (which are positively charged) the body doesn't need without trapping vital mineral nutrients like calcium, zinc,

* ACIMD (American Center for Integrative Medicine and Dentistry) Training Seminar notes (Boulder, CO, June 2015).

and magnesium that the body does need. And they're remarkably low cost—especially compared to many aspects of contemporary medicine—and have virtually no downside when used properly.

Removing heavy metals (such as mercury) from the body can be a significant step toward improved whole-body health. Because zeolites trap the higher-positively charged toxins, your body doesn't need them to leave the "good stuff" alone, and they can be a valuable addition to detoxification procedures. The long-term results of detoxification using this method can be very beneficial. The process, however, is not a quick one and requires patience in the patient. It can take up to several months to accomplish chelation that brings toxic metal levels down to acceptable amounts.*

So, what are some good chelation products you can use? I've outlined below several good ones, along with a few details about their use.

1. Advanced Cellular Zeolite (ACZ nano, extra strength) from Results DNA.
   - Contains high concentrations of clinoptilolite zeolite per dose, which indicates the quality of the product.
   - Removes fluorine and chlorine in an intraoral spray delivery system. This is important because fluorine and chlorine are strong oxidizing agents that contribute to the aging process; remember, they are electron stealers.
   - Detoxifies blood cells, balances pH levels, and *reverses* acute chemical and allergic reactions.
   - Increases urinary Hg (mercury) output up to 103,500 percent over baseline during a twelve-hour test period. (Talk about a good way to get mercury out of your system.)
   - Excretion is through the urinary tract, a highly efficient way to remove waste. Irreversibly binds and removes heavy metal toxins, radioactive toxins, volatile organic compounds (VOCs), and free radicals of all types. Does not bind to macro-minerals like IV-chelation.

2. Zeolites for detoxification
   - Developed by chelation therapy expert Dr. Gary Gordon.
   - An oral zeolite, which is an especially effective form.
   - Another newer zeolite product is advanced TRS by Coseva.

* Medical News Today, What To Know About Chelation Therapy, https://www.medicalnewstoday.com/articles/chelation-therapy.

3. NCD, Natural Cellular Defense by Waiora
    - This is an MLM product that you must sign up to use but it's well worth doing.
    - Recommended use: seven to twelve months. I've had several patients on this product with good results.

The Amazing Benefits of Oil Pulling[*, †]

Ayurvedic medicine is a medical system consisting of the application of herbs, diet, and massage first developed more than three thousand years ago in India. Among its many holistic approaches to healing, one of its treatment protocols in particular—oil pulling—is especially applicable to oral healing. The protocol uses coconut oil or sesame seed oil to draw toxins out of inflamed gingival tissues, and the oil's antibacterial, antiviral, and antifungal characteristics make it useful for treating a wide variety of oral health conditions.

So, how does oil pulling work? When you have inflammation or an infection in your mouth, cell-signaling compounds called cytokines are produced by your liver. These inflammatory cytokines tell your inflammatory system that your body is "on fire" and turns on a transcription switch called NF-kB, or Nuclear Factor-kappa Beta. This starts the process of elevated chronic inflammation and represents the beginning of chronic degenerative disease (CDD).

Your mouth is home to billions of bacteria, yeast, and viruses—some good, some not-so-good. This is called the oral microbiome. These bugs can travel around and override the cellular barriers designed to protect you from infection. The first signs of trouble are red, inflamed, and bleeding gums. Next is periodontal disease that can affect your heart, lungs, and all of your major organ systems. It can even negatively impact pregnancy.

From your mouth, these bugs can enter your bloodstream through the gingival sulcus barrier in your gums and wreak havoc by causing inflammation in the inner layer of your blood vessels, called the endothelium. When this happens, your immune system goes into overdrive. But as bad as the problem is, it can be improved by using oil pulling.

This ancient detoxification protocol pulls toxins out of your gum tissues and teeth (including failed root canal infections and the like). It can even reduce problems with plaque biofilms by making them less sticky.

There are numerous benefits to oil pulling:

1. Fresher, better breath and less decay, especially in children.
2. Decreasing oral, gingival, and periodontal infections.

---

* Ketabi, *Ayurveda*.

† Claire Ragozzino, *Living Ayurveda: Oil Pulling and Tongue Scraping* (Roost Books, 2020), 50.

3. Decreasing non-beneficial oral bacteria, along with decreasing systemic infections and disease.
4. Decreasing oral inflammation, a.k.a. gingivitis and bleeding gums.
5. Decreasing cardiovascular disease (CVD).
6. A healthier, less active immune system, with fewer colds.
7. A healthier, better functioning probiotic bacterial ratio by increasing the beneficial bacteria.

How and when should you use oil pulling?

- Oil-pull for 10 to 20 minutes in the morning, using a teaspoon or two of either sesame or coconut oil or a mixture of both and swish it around in your mouth, then spit the oil in the trash (not the sink—it will harden in the pipes and clog your drain). Do not swallow the oil. An advantage of using coconut oil is that it is a medium chain triglyceride (MCT) which kills candida, and it's a healthy fat.
- Brush with Pearl Nature's Toothpaste®. Its superior ingredients will remineralize teeth and raise nitric oxide levels.
- Add twenty-one drops ConcenTrace® Mineral Drops into water or juice, along with seven to ten drops Pearl Silica Drops® (three to five drops for children). This raises the voltage in all of your cellular membranes, plus many other benefits for your teeth and bones.
- Rinse with food-grade hydrogen peroxide.
- You can also rinse with baking soda, as this increases the alkalinity in your mouth. Remember to keep the pH at or above 7.0, thereby decreasing plaque, dental biofilm, and decay!

How to Clean Your Teeth Naturally

As you might imagine, at our naturopathic and holistic dentistry center, one of the most frequently asked questions is "What's the best way to clean my teeth?"

So, I've come up with a quick list of to-dos:

1. Oil pulling and tongue scraping.
2. You may not be able to brush after every time you eat, but you can rinse your mouth with water. I highly recommend that you do this. Swish, then spit. This dilutes the oral acids.
3. Drink one eight-ounce glass of pure water daily with freshly squeezed lemon juice. Add back the minerals (ConcenTrace® *Minerals Drops* and Pearl Silica Drops®). Do this three times daily. I recommend drinking four ounces of mineralized water every half hour during the waking hours. Your system can handle the smaller amounts more efficiently.
4. Use a Sonicare toothbrush with baking soda, coconut oil, and Pearl Nature's Toothpaste®.

5. If you chew gum or must eat sugar, then use xylitol, but even then, use them sparingly. And never, ever drink soda pop—it's poison, plain and simple (follow the safe sugars list).
6. Follow my 80 percent anti-inflammatory foods list (in the appendix).
7. Use ConcenTrace® Mineral Drops daily—twenty-one drops per day, along with six to ten Pearl Silica Drops®, adjusted for bowel tolerance—especially for children (three to five drops).

You can augment the effectiveness of these good cleaning practices with these overall healthy patterns:

1. Keep your mouth slightly alkaline—a pH above 7.0 is the best. (Below 5.5 starts the decay process.)
2. Keep your macro- and micro-mineral content high.
3. Use essential oils daily, especially clove and Thieves® oil.
4. Use ozonated oil and ozonated water.
5. Consume a ketogenic diet, or a mostly plant-based diet, and especially stay away from all refined sugars.
6. Control your oral probiotic content by using *Streptococcus salivarius* K-12 and M-18.
7. Stay away from commercial toothpastes that are loaded with toxic ingredients like fluoride and sodium lauryl sulphate (foaming agent).*
8. Use proper breath management by breathing deeply through your nose while keeping your mouth closed, as this limits the drying effect of air, and increases oxygen intake to the lungs.
9. Maintain good hydration by drinking half your body weight in ounces of water every day.
10. Take Liposomal Vitamin C and Glutathione daily to help detox.

Remember: Detoxification is a lifelong process, *not* a seven- to twenty-one-day deal.

A Special Word about Your Baby's Teeth

Another question I hear frequently is: "When should I bring my baby in to see you?" Patients also wonder about tooth eruption patterns, arch development, fluoride, teething, sealants, dental decay, healthy nutrition, and remineralization.†

* International Society for Fluoride Research, Budapest Study, 21st Congress Budapest, Hungary.

† Dr. Thomas Lokensgard, *Patients Guide to Remineralization of Teeth and Bone*, Protocol, https://www.drlokensgard.com/shop.

All of these are important questions for the development of babies' teeth because baby teeth are essential for:*

- Proper digestive function
- Proper speech development
- Proper support of the developing permanent dentition (i.e., holding orthodontic space)
- Development of self-esteem and social skills, proper lip support, and a positive lower facial profile
- Proper nutrition, allowing the gut to absorb food efficiently
- Correct placement of the mandibular condyles (jaw growth)

Here are my recommendations on care for baby teeth:

- **Teething.** You can apply OxyMist® to the affected area of the gums to help alleviate pain. You can also use *Arnica montana*, hypericum, or clove oil. Never use Tylenol, it blocks glutathione.
- **Dental arch development.** It's important to monitor facial growth and development early on, starting around age three. We correct parafunctional habits as soon as they are identified. This includes cross-bites, deficient airways, deficient dental arches, and tongue-ties, to name a few.
- **Eruption patterns.** Patterns and time of eruption for children can vary enormously, so don't worry about the timing or sequencing. Look at dental arch size instead, but begin brushing babies' teeth as soon as they erupt. Also look for a high-vaulted palate, narrow arch form, overlapping of the upper teeth, or the retrusion of the chin profile. (Deep bite)
- **Dental sealants.** Avoid them, unless ozone is used first.
- **Mercury fillings.**† Never, never, never let any dentist put mercury fillings in your child's teeth, ever.
- **Bring baby to the dentist as soon as you see the eruption of teeth.** Lower centrals are usually the first teeth you will see.
- **Fluoride.** Don't do it. It's not necessary, and it disrupts thyroid function by displacing iodine.
- **Breastfeed your baby.** There are too many advantages of breastfeeding to mention them all, but here are the top three:
  1. It will give your newborn the needed probiotic support for healthy GI development. The gut is where 70 percent of the immune system resides, and breastfed babies produce higher levels of antibodies and have fewer infections.

---

* Weston A. Price Foundation; *WAPF Journal*, Fall 2017.

† IAOMT, Mercury Poisoning, https://iaomt.org/resources/dental-mercury-facts/mercury-poisoning-symptoms-dental-amalgam/.

2. Essential fatty acids and correct EPA/DHA ratios are necessary for proper brain support. Mother's milk contains the correct ratio of these needed healthy fats. Think of this as baby's essential brain fuel.
3. The suckling action during breastfeeding helps to properly develop lower jaw structure, and it contributes to proper growth of the lower face by positioning the jaw down and forward. Look for a tongue-tie. If baby's tongue cannot reach his or her palate, then there is a problem.

What's Good for You? Serum Compatibility Testing

While there are no perfect dental materials, some are much less immunologically reactive than others. Serum compatibility testing (SCT) is one way to find out which dental materials are best for you. SCT is a blood serum test that determines how reactive the dental materials placed in your mouth may be to your immune system. The test measures your immunoglobulins (proteins), which may possibly react to the dental materials in your mouth and tells just how reactive the materials might be.

Not everyone needs this kind of testing, but a SCT should be performed if you have multiple chemical sensitivities or are severely immune-compromised.

A couple of the testing companies I recommend are Clifford Consulting and Bio Comp. The test costs around $300. It will tell you which bio-reactive dental materials are best for you.

Here are some of the dental materials known to be less bio-reactive: Show this list to your dentistry team.

- Diamond Lite, composite material
- Diamond Crown, composite material
- Ora MD, an all-natural mouth rinse
- Our new toothpaste (this replenishes calcium and phosphate in the saliva which is good for remineralization)
- Low-fusing porcelain, e-max porcelain onlays
- ASEA, a redox-signaling supplement for vital cellular communication
- MCHA, microcrystalline hydroxyapatite for bone support and remodeling for healthier bone mineral density. It's in our Pearl Nature's Toothpaste®.
- Cal Apatite, with magnesium
- Ostera, contains selective kinase response modulators
- IPS-e max, low-fusing porcelain
- Thera-Cal, calcium hydroxide liner
- Voco products, composites, cements, and others
- Argentyn23®, a nano-silver antibiotic that kills lots of pathogenic bugs
- Colostrum, has high levels of Secretory-IgA immunoglobulins to boost immunity. Bovine colostrum is also suitable.

- Iodine, used to decrease capsular contraction in breast augmentation and also used in treatment of periodontal disease. Iodine has also been shown to balance your pH and flush out fluoride.
- White oak bark
- White willow bark, anticavity and antimicrobial, plus a painkiller
- Black walnut, anticavity and antimicrobial
- Coenzyme Q10, especially for periodontal and cardiac conditions
- Biodentine, a biocompatible dentin liner
- Photocore, buildup material

We've covered a lot of ground so far, and I hope you now get the picture of what good health should look like. But since most of us don't start with good health, let's look next at some truly healthy solutions for TMJ Dysfunction.

CHAPTER 6

A Little TLC for the TMJ

As we've talked about your mouth as the window to your health, we've focused primarily on teeth, gums, and the structures *inside* your mouth. One area that deserves its own brief chapter is the TMJs. The temporomandibular joints (TMJs) have their own unique impact on a person's health. In fact, if they're not working correctly, the TMJs can be ruinous for a person's quality of life.

WHAT IS TMJ DISORDER?

Many people, even doctors, nurses, and insurance companies, use the term TMJ. But what does this abbreviation mean? The term TMJ is an abbreviation for temporomandibular joint, or the jaw joint. In fact, there are really two TMJs, one directly in front of each ear.

The TMJ is the joint formed by the temporal bone of the skull (temporo) with the lower jaw or mandible (hence, mandibular). These joints move each time we chew, talk, or even swallow. The TMJ is actually a sliding joint, not a ball and socket like the shoulder. This sliding allows for pressures placed on the joint to be distributed throughout the joint and not just focused in one area.

The TMJs are the most complex joints in the human body. Placed between these two bones is a disc, just like the one between your vertebrae, called the articular disc. This disc is primarily made of cartilage and in the TMJ acts like a third bone. The disc, being attached to a muscle, actually moves with certain movements of the TMJ.

The nerve to the TMJ is a branch of the trigeminal nerve and therefore, an injury to the TMJ may be confused with neuralgia of the trigeminal nerve. The two bones of the TMJs are held together by a series of ligaments, any of which can be damaged, just like any other joint.

A damaged TMJ ligament usually results in a dislocation of the disc, the lower jaw, or both. Also, the bones are connected by two main muscles—the temporalis and the masseter—and a muscle just discovered by Dr. Wesley Shankland called the zygo-mandibular. Any or all of these muscles may be painful and produce pain in the TMJ or at the very least, abnormal movement of the lower jaw.

TMJ problems manifest in unexpected ways also. They can trigger pain in the shoulders and back due to muscular contraction, a condition called myofascial pain dysfunction syndrome. Some people who suffer with TMJ problems experience dizziness, disorientation, headaches, ringing in the ears (tinnitus), clicking, popping, and even joints that lock open or closed as a result. If you are experiencing some of these symptoms, a self-check will help determine whether you have reason to think your TMJs may be the problem.

In Appendix 4, I've provided a twenty-five-question self-evaluation you can use to decide whether you should seek professional help for a TMJ problem.

Self-Care for Temporomandibular Muscle and Joint Disorders

- **Apply moist heat or cold to the joint or muscles that are sore.** Heat or ice applications, used up to four times per day, can reduce joint or muscle pain and relax the muscles. For heat, warm a wet towel for approximately 1 minute. You then wrap this moist towel around a hot-water bottle or heated gel pack to keep it warm longer. Apply it to the affected area for fifteen to twenty minutes. For cold, use ice wrapped in a thin cloth. At first, you may feel a burning sensation, which is normal. Keep ice on the painful area no more than five minutes after you feel some numbness. Use what feels best but in general, heat is used for more chronic pain conditions, and cold for acute conditions.

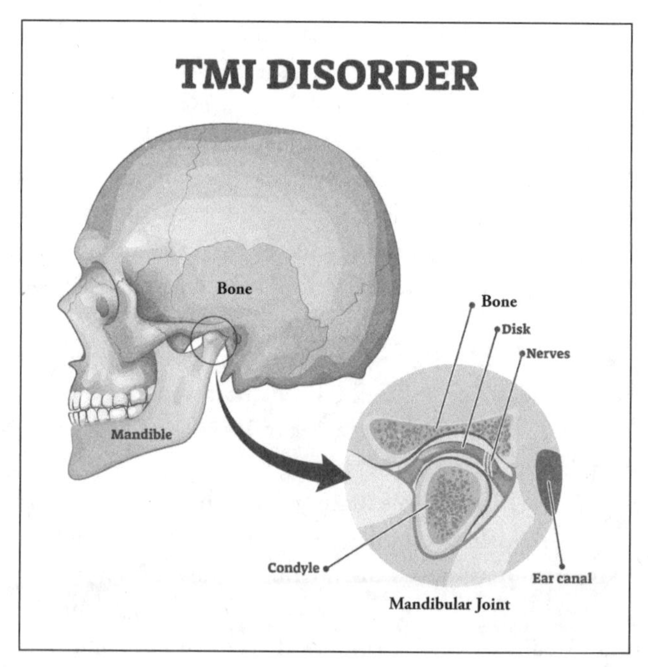

Illustration of temporomandibular joint disorder (TMJ). Credit: VectorMine.

- **Eat a pain-free diet.** Avoid hard foods, such as French bread or bagels. Avoid chewy food such as steak. Cut fruits and steamed vegetables into small pieces. Do not chew gum.
- **Keep your tongue up, teeth apart, and jaw muscles relaxed.** Closely monitor your jaw position during waking hours so that you maintain your jaw in a relaxed, comfortable position. This often involves placing your tongue lightly on the palate behind your upper front teeth (find this position by saying "n"), allowing the teeth to be apart while relaxing the jaw muscles.
- **Avoid oral habits and activities that put strain on the jaw and neck.** Oral habits such as teeth clenching, teeth grinding (bruxism), teeth touching or resting together, biting cheeks or lips, tongue pushing against teeth, jaw tensing, biting objects, shoulder shrugging, neck tensing, and other activities such as yawning, resting your jaw on your hand, or over-chewing. If noticed, these habits should be replaced with positive habits in a tongue-up position.
- **Keep your head up, chin in, and shoulders up and back.** Closely monitor your head position over your shoulders to maintain a balance, relax your head, neck, and shoulder muscles without a forward head posture. This will help to reduce strain to jaw, neck, and shoulder muscles.
- **Learn and practice relaxation and abdominal breathing.** This will help reduce your reactions to stressful life events and decrease tension in the jaw and neck, increase HRV, and parasympathetic nervous system function.
- **Identify the events that trigger the pain.** Use a pain diary to review daily activities that aggravate the pain and modify your behavior accordingly.
- **Get a good night's sleep.** Manage your sleep environment. Reduce light and noise and sleep on a comfortable mattress, avoiding sleeping on your stomach. Reduce stimulating activities in late evening including computer work and exercising.
- **Avoid caffeine.** Caffeine and caffeine-like drugs, such as coffee, tea, soda, power drinks, and chocolate, can interfere with sleep and increase muscle tension. Some decaffeinated coffee has up to half as much caffeine as regular coffee. The bolder the roast, the less the caffeine.
- **Use anti-inflammatory and pain-reducing medications for the short term only.** Over-the-counter ibuprofen, naproxen, or aspirin can reduce joint and muscle pain, along with arnica, hypericum or Sam-e. Never use Tylenol, as it blocks glutathione production. This is bad news.

Bruxism, Grinding, Malocclusion, and Mineral Deficiency*

Bad bites, called malocclusions, are related to abnormal muscle function and related to the cardiovascular system via its effect on heart rate variability (HRV). How? HRV is a measure of the proper functioning of the parasympathetic nervous system (PSNS), a division of the autonomic nervous system (ANS). This is your "relax, sleep, and digest" nervous system. Ask your healthcare practitioner to test your HRV.

The other component or division of the ANS is the sympathetic nervous system (SNS), or your "fight and flight" nervous system. These two systems must be balanced.

A high level of HRV is most desirable, and a low functioning level of HRV is undesirable. HRV is further related to many physiological functions including:

- Bruxism (grinding) decreases HRV, and can also be related to magnesium deficiency.
- Cancer decreases HRV and signals huge problems.
- Airway obstruction (OSA) also decreases HRV and signals O_2 metabolism problems.
- Unbalanced jaw position or malocclusions cause decreased HRV.
- Inflammation is increased by a decreasing HRV.
- Increasing mercury levels and increasing toxicity lowers HRV and raises BP.
- TMD issues decrease HRV.
- Proper breathing techniques also improve HRV.
- Earthing has a positive effect on PVCs and HRV.†
- MRAs and ortho-tropics can improve and increase HRV.

These are inverse relationships. Remember, a low HRV means that the SNS is spiking. This is not a good scenario.

* Jeffrey S. Hindin, DDS; IAOMT, Conference Lecture Notes (Las Vegas, NV, September 2017).

† Stephen Sinatra, MD, et al., *Earthing* (Basic Health Publications, Inc.; 2nd edition, 2014).

CHAPTER 7

The War on Inflammation

If the treatment is killing your patient, then stop the treatment.
—Charles Krauthammer, MD

The most important starting point for health education and combating disease is to grasp—and deal with—the significance of silent inflammation. Just how significant is it to begin with this focus? In a nutshell, silent inflammation is, quite simply, the newest, most dramatic measure of disease available.

Chronic inflammation is the result of decreased metabolism and decreased oxygen use, which decreases energy production and produces less ATP. Think of fatigue. Frank Shallenberger, MD, a mentor of mine, proclaimed at his most recent medical conference, "There is but one disease, genetics aside, and that is aging." I believe he hit the nail squarely on its head.

Breaking the Silence

Biochemist, author, and creator of the Zone diet, Barry Sears, PhD, explained succinctly in a 2007 A4M lecture what silent inflammation is and how it affects us: "Silent inflammation, is a condition that occurs when the body's natural immune response goes awry. It's been linked to heart disease, cancer, diabetes, even dementia and other health threats; and it can go on for years, undetected."

The paradigm shift to the silent inflammatory disease model is the centerpiece of integrative medical and dental treatment. There is a cytoplasmic transcription switch called NF-k-Beta which gets turned on when inflammatory mediators trigger it. We've all experienced some form of obvious inflammation at one time or another—a small wound gets infected then turns red, something irritates our gums, and they become inflamed. These external examples, though, are only a small part of the inflammation story, and actually examples that show that something good can happen with inflammation. Inflammation is a necessary part of the healing process, but when it kicks into overdrive, it results in disease instead of healing. In that case, it becomes a silent killer much like high blood pressure or diabetes.

The hidden aspect of inflammation is what makes it so dangerous. And to make matters worse, we are generally unaware of what causes this condition. Let me begin by showing you the astounding array of issues we face that cause the problem in the first place. We'll get into detail about the causes and what to do about silent inflammation.

Here is a "laundry list" of things we all face almost every day that can lead to silent inflammation:

- Toxic and or polluted water
- Trans-fatty foods
- Electromagnetic radiation (EMFs)
- Chronic stress
- Indoor air pollution
- Heavy metal toxicity, especially mercury fillings
- All pharmaceutical drugs
- Automobile exhaust
- Cigarette smoke
- Alcohol
- Fast foods
- UV radiation
- Pesticides, xenoestrogens
- Viruses, fungi, EBV, pseudomonas, spirochetes, bacteria, COVID virus, etc.
- Insecticides
- Preservatives and pthalates, plastics
- Low hormone levels
- Not enough sleep
- Eating too much GMO food or food that contains glyphosates
- Vaccinations
- Bleeding gums
- Periodontal disease
- Failed root canals

And I've saved the worst for last. The greatest culprit of all is the standard American diet—often referred to, quite accurately, as the SAD diet.

When you consider all the factors arrayed against your efforts to enjoy good health, it can be daunting.

Yet winning the battle for a healthful lifestyle is completely doable. So, let's drill down on how to defeat silent inflammation in your life.

"You cannot pharmacologically intoxicate a person into health."
—David Baltimore, MD, ND

I have patients who are on fourteen different medications. So, here's my question: How is one supposed to get well if he or she is on fourteen different synthetic medications? Often one medication is required to counteract the side effects of the first one which then requires another to counteract the effects of the second, and so on. Take Protonix or Nexium, for example. These are acid blockers and in most cases of heartburn, that is the wrong approach. Why? Because as we age, we produce less stomach acid, not more!

The result is a shutdown of acid production in your gut and an epidemic of overprescription of medication (polypharmacy) and little true health to show for it. The body simply becomes dependent on the infusion of synthetic (none of which are biologic) pharmaceutical chemicals to mask symptoms of disease rather than solving the disease problem itself. Remember this: all pharmaceutical drugs are acidic and therefore inflammatory.

So, here's my question to you: Is your body designed to run on nutrition or on Big Pharma drugs? The pharmaceutical industry and its misguided TV commercials would have you believe in the magic bullet theory of healthcare. In their scenario, you get sick, take a pill, mask the symptoms, and live symptom-free ever after. But how's that working for the millions of people who don't take just one pill or two, but are chronically on multiple medications? This is what I'm referring to as the polypharmacy merry-go-round. There is no magic bullet for good health.

We've been programmed, however, to think there is such a thing. Truth, though, is stronger, more vibrant, and ultimately more healing than to continue abiding by a dysfunctional fiction. The real answer is integrative medicine and functional dentistry.

Notice I didn't say the *easy* answer. In the face of the countless physical, mental, and spiritual influences to the contrary, it's not easy to focus on developing a lifestyle of genuine health. This is especially true because we've been taught to think of good health as something doctors provide us through our annual checkups, not something we do for ourselves day in and day out. But the same is true in dentistry. A six-month checkup is not the be-all and end-all. In fact, there isn't any clinical relevance to it at all.

I was at a large dental conference a few years back, when the speaker asked if anyone was aware of the historical beginnings of the six-month dental checkup. I was sitting toward the back of the room and announced to the person next to me, rather loudly, "Bucky Beaver!" The speaker looked toward me and asked, "Who said that?" I somewhat sheepishly raised my hand as he exclaimed, "You are correct!" He proceeded: here is how the insurance industry embraced the six-month cleaning protocol, better known as the Bucky Beaver story.

In the 1950s, there was a brand of toothpaste called Ipana toothpaste that had a mascot named Bucky Beaver who told everyone to "Brush your teeth after every meal and visit your dentist twice a year." This became the insurance industry standard of clinical care in dentistry.

There is no clinical evidence or relevance at all. The truth is that some of you need dental care at three-, four-, seven-, twelve-, or twenty-four- to thirty-six-month intervals. Some of you need X-rays at varying intervals, also. It's really what you do on a daily basis that creates excellent dental health as well as incorporating the principles on the rest of these pages. In addition, we've also been told that we can safely eat the stuff sold in our grocery stores because, "certainly the government wouldn't let them sell it to us if it were bad." Right? Wrong.

If you want to be healthy, I'd estimate you should bypass at least 80 percent of what you see on the grocery store shelves (maybe only 60 percent if you shop at a natural foods store). How do you know which 20 percent is okay for your health? Good question, but first, let's look at the other obstacles in the path of good health—and how to get past them.

Health Education: The Prescription for Disease Prevention

Earlier, I quoted Hippocrates, the famous Greek physician who lived more than twenty centuries ago. He was amazingly prescient for his time, and that's why he's still worthy of being quoted. Since then—and especially in the past century—science has revealed an astounding level of intricacy as to how we function, and that has added immeasurably to how well we should be able to handle medical problems today. We have tremendous advantages in knowledge that Hippocrates did not have, but the knowledge has to be put to work in beneficial ways.

Today, in medicine and dentistry, we are moving away from the theory (the excuse) that chronic degenerative disease (CDD) is caused mainly by genetics. We now know that CDD is caused primarily (80 percent) by lifestyle, improper nutrients, and lack of proper metabolism driven by lowered oxygen consumption caused by improper breathing through your mouth. Just because you have a genetic predisposition does not mean you need to express it, phenotypically. This is very good news and is why lifestyle, nutrigenomics, and epigenetics are so critically important.*

There's a lot to know—which is what acquiring health knowledge is all about.

There was a time when the science of physics established by Sir Isaac Newton seemed like the gold standard of understanding the laws of motion, et al. His principles reigned supreme for several hundred years until Albert Einstein blew everyone's minds with his discovery of relativity and the corresponding physics. Still, the combination of Newtonian physics and Einsteinian physics has a lot to teach us about how the physical world operates.

Newton and Einstein provide an analogy of traditional medicine (Newtonian) and cellular energy-based medicine (Einsteinian). By using the newest body of knowledge, we can create a medical model for your health and genetic and

---

* Kendall Stewart, MD, Genomix Conference (Houston, TX, 2016).

wellness optimization. As a result, we can live healthier, more vibrant lives. God created us as biochemical beings as well as bioenergetic beings.

A well-rounded and productive education on health, then, includes a focus on the following:

- Oral inflammation and total oral fitness
- Oral biology and dental infections
- Sleep and airway control
- Brain and neurotransmitter balance
- Systemic inflammatory control and immune function improvement
- Digestive health and maintenance
- Stress control and proper sleep, NEI Axis control
- Targeted nutraceutical support, which increases proper enzyme function
- Combating chronic degenerative disease
- Bioidentical hormone therapy
- Nutrition and weight control
- Improving muscle mass and balance
- Cardiovascular balance and mitochondrial biogenesis

Altogether, these approaches to health dramatically reduce the risk of:

- Cancer
- Heart disease
- Osteoporosis
- Memory loss
- Mood dysfunction
- Digestive dysbiosis
- Growing old before your time

Since I'm a naturopathic, antiaging dentist, you might not be surprised to hear me say that our examination of inflammation begins in the mouth. Part of my own journey was to observe that much of what I saw in a patient's mouth reflected their overall well-being. And now I know why—and want you to know, too.

Inflammation can be easily detected in the oral cavity (mouth, nasal passages, and adjoining structures) with oral bio-inflammation cytokine testing. Cytokine testing measures your inflammatory markers to determine your level of inflammation. Surprisingly, your saliva reveals enough about your lymphatic functions that we can use it instead of blood for this sort of testing. And this is good news because most people prefer giving a salivary sample to being poked by a needle for a blood test.

Antiaging practitioners can administer this kind of test to give you a benchmark for your level of inflammation. The age-old worn-out "standard of care" is the testing and "blood work" that insurance companies will pay for, as long as there is a *condition and symptom* attached to the claim so they can provide you with a prescription drug that is anything but biological. The goal here is to diminish the symptom.

Before engaging in formal testing, though, you can make your own personal assessment of where you stand. If you do an informal evaluation first, it can help you decide whether lab testing is needed to determine just how severe the inflammation has become in your particular situation.

A good place to start is Laird Wellness who has three options for blood panels and consultations and coaching services.* Scott Laird, ND, is also a wealth of information with his podcasts and videos.†

Read through the list of ten conditions or lifestyle practices that contribute significantly to silent inflammation and see how many are affecting you.

1. You're overweight (the greater the weight, the greater the inflammatory problem).
2. You use birth control pills.
3. You take beta blockers or diuretics. You're on statin drugs or other cholesterol-lowering drugs.
4. You have multiple failed root canals, mercury fillings, jaw cavitations, and multiple dental infections.
5. You're sleep deprived or have obstructive sleep apnea (OSA).
6. You suffer with chronic fatigue (more than 50 percent of my patients check this on their med history form).
7. Your fingernails are brittle.
8. You are routinely groggy upon waking up or you are a mouth breather.
9. You crave carbohydrates and salty foods and are mineral deficient.
10. You're dehydrated, meaning, you don't drink enough water (emphasis on water—soft drinks, coffee, and other beverages don't count). Your water must be mineralized and clean.

If you are concerned because you see yourself in a number of the items in the list (even one of them can cause problems), let me give you one quick and enjoyable way to begin your winning lifestyle. The anti-inflammatory lifestyle (eating, drinking, good habits, etc.) works because it increases natural killer cells (NK cells).‡

---

* Scott Laird, ND, Laird Wellness, http://www.lairdwellness.com.

† AHealthAwakening, http://www.youtube.com/results?search_query=the+health+awakening+scott+laird and https://rumble.com/c/c-1158311.

‡ A4M 14th Annual International Congress on Anti-Aging Medicine Intensive Workshops /Certification Programs (Las Vegas, NV, December 7–9, 2006).

And the fun part is that some studies have shown that something we can all do more of actually increases natural killer cell function. This boosts your immune system. You want to know what that is? It's smiling and laughing. The more you smile and laugh, the more you help your body combat silent inflammation. So, start smiling and laughing, and read on about what else you can do.

The Fat Factor

Inflammation is driven largely by what you eat, and a key component of the plan is to reduce inflammatory fat in your diet. It would not be overstating the case by much to say that the popular media view of fat intake and what causes obesity is all wrong. That's because it's based on an overly simplistic pseudo-understanding that goes something like this: "If you eat something that has fat in it, it makes you fat."

The real process is not nearly so simple. To give you the real scoop though, I'll have to explain a bit about a topic that may sound intimidating, but hang with me. You'll need to know a little about dietary endocrinology.

Endocrinology is the science of the chemical modulators your body produces known as hormones. They manage almost everything that happens inside you. These are your informational messengers. Dietary endocrinology, then, is the study of how what you eat affects your hormone production.

The food you eat produces a hormonal response that results in either the production of insulin, glucagon, and/or eicosanoids. These are three of the hormones I'm referring to. What's important here is the role of the eicosanoid hormones. These are what you might call super hormones that control all of your other hormones, and they exist in every cell in your body. The type of fat you eat changes the balance of eicosanoids. This is a really big deal.[*]

There are two types of fats: inflammatory and noninflammatory. Omega-6 fats are inflammatory, and they trigger the release of arachidonic acid (AA). This is bad news. It is the inflammatory pathway. On the other hand, omega-3 fats are anti-inflammatory, and they protect you from chronic inflammation. All omega-6 fats are high in arachidonic acid (inflammatory), so, for example, all vegetable oils in the grocery store are inflammatory.

So, one quick change you can make for better health is to stop using all cheap-o vegetable oils, especially canola oil. There are omega-3, omega-6, omega-7, and omega-9 fatty acid oils, and the ratio of omega-3 to omega-6 oils should ideally be one-to-one. In America, the ratio can be as high as twenty to 1, omega-6, to omega-3. No wonder we're so inflamed. The correct omega fats kept in the correct ratio control silent inflammation, not to mention prevent heart attacks.[†, ‡]

---

* A4M, 14th Annual International Congress on Anti-Aging Medicine.

† ANA (American Nutraceutical Association) Conference and Journal 8, 2005.

‡ Floyd H. Chilton, PhD, *Inflammation Nation* (Atria Books, 2006).

The problem we all face is that the standard American diet does a great job of increasing arachidonic acid (think "inflammation"), the inflammatory pathway. Your body tries to sequester the AA in order to neutralize it. And guess how it sequesters AA? By increasing the volume of your fat cells, known as adipocytes, with water. This is a major cause of obesity as it sets off a chain of inflammatory reactions that ultimately results in insulin resistance, another key cause of obesity.

This type of inflammation is caused by sugar. Lots of it. Now back to inflammatory fat. What began in the body as a sequestering of toxic fat in order to protect your body from unwanted AA ends up causing severe consequences of inflammation and obesity because we were never designed to have to deal with so many omega-6 fatty acids and so much sugar.

The body considers inflammation so toxic that it is set up to gain weight by increasing the volume of fat cells rather than to allow inflammation to run rampant. Fat is a natural biological defense against inflammation. It's the omega-6 fatty acids that are making you inflamed, fat, and sick. Sugar also, especially the refined type, which drives up insulin signaling and causes you to store the excess sugar as triglycerides, thus increasing your fat deposits even further.

So, what are you supposed to do? Manage what you put in your mouth. Learn to better understand nutrigenomics, epigenetics, and dietary endocrinology and how what you eat affects your hormone levels.

Anti-Inflammatory Eating

Here are some tips for anti-inflammatory eating with examples of popular eating plans:

- Intermittent fasting
- Forks over Knives—Dr. Esselstyn's whole-food, plant-based lifestyle approach
- The Zone diet—a moderate carb diet great for decreasing silent inflammation
- The Hollywood Cookie Diet—JUST KIDDING!
- The PAN Asian Mediterranean diet
- The GAPS diet
- The Weston A. Price diet
- The paleo diet
- The ketogenic diet
- The plant-based diet

On the other side is the standard American diet (SAD)—an ultra-processed, bioengineered high-carb diet that causes increased insulin and fat storage and is highly inflammatory.

A problem arises, though, with referring to these—or any particular pattern of eating—as a "diet." Although the Greek root word from which we derive the term "diet" means "a way of life," we tend to associate the idea of a diet with "dieting." And dieting triggers the idea that the particular pattern of eating is a temporary plan, which, after a goal is reached (usually weight loss), the pattern will be abandoned.

The standard definition of a diet in America is a three-month binge starvation plan so you can fit into a bathing suit. This is not a very effective long-term plan. For that reason, I prefer not to refer to an anti-inflammatory eating pattern as a "diet." I'd rather have you think of it as a complete lifestyle change, and in that regard, there are fairly simple guidelines as to how to create an anti-inflammatory lifestyle for yourself:

1. Use intermittent fasting (eat only between the hours of 12 p.m. and 7 p.m.).
2. Have some protein during that time, in the right balance with carbohydrates. This is called link and balance dieting.
3. Consume primarily low-glycemic fruits and vegetables.
4. Incorporate healthy oils such as omega-3, MCT (coconut oil), and olive oil.
5. Caloric restriction (CR)—eat less. Eating too much causes oxidative stress and taxes your kidneys. It is your kidneys that must deal with an incomplete protein burn. Plus, with today's food costs it's a whole lot cheaper.
6. Start by skipping breakfast. Studies show that people who skip breakfast tend to become healthier over time. This is intermittent fasting.
7. Don't drink water with your meal—especially cold water as this reduces the hydrochloric acid (HCl) content in your stomach. A naturopathic principle.

THE GLYCEMIC INDEX (GI) and GLYCEMIC LOAD (GL)

The GI is a system of measuring the body's response to equal portions of foods with carbohydrates such as bread, pasta, rice, fruits, peas, beans, yogurt, milk, and vegetables. The higher the number, the greater the blood sugar response and therefore the harder the body has to work to bring that blood sugar down. So, a low-GI food that causes a negligible rise in blood sugar is a healthier food to eat than one that has a high GI. Generally, a GI greater than 70 is considered to be high, a GI of 50 to 69 is medium, and a GI of 50 or less is relatively low.

Because the GI is calculated for a food portion containing 50 grams of carbohydrate, the resulting number may be a little deceptive. Carrots are a good example; to eat 50 grams of carbohydrate in carrots would mean eating over 1 pound—or about five large carrots. Very few people would do that. The GL was developed, which is a more meaningful and realistic way to assess the true impact of a carbohydrate food. The GL is based on the GI but further develops the concept by taking into account the amount of carbohydrates in one serving.*

Foods that have a low GI almost always have a low GL. But foods with an intermediate or high GI may range from low to high GL—it all depends on the suggested serving size. This may explain why many people who are professional dieters think that carrots or peas are too high in sugar. While the GI for both falls in the moderate range, their actual GL is 3. Watermelon with its high GI of 72 has a low GL of 4 due to the low carbohydrate content in a ¾ cup serving. Even if you were to eat double that amount, which is quite possible, you are still eating less than a GL of 10 for that food (which is still in the low GL range).

THE GLYCEMIC INDEX

- 50 or less is low glycemic
- 50–70 is moderately glycemic
- 70 or higher is high glycemic

The late Dr. Shari Lieberman came up with a succinct list of benefits of consuming a low-glycemic diet. I was very fortunate to have studied under her. Here, in her own words, are the benefits and her thoughts on the low-glycemic index:

- To control weight, inflammation, and body composition.
- We were designed to eat a low-glycemic diet.
- Traditional diets have low glycemic indexes.
- High-glycemic contents throw the metabolic switch to store fat (this increases insulin).
- We were not genetically engineered to tolerate massive swings in glucose or sucrose.
- GI is a measurement of the impact of carbohydrates on *blood sugar* levels crucial to proper internal balance.
- There is no calorie counting or restriction required.
- Caloric restriction (CR) slows your basal metabolic rate (BMR) by as much as 10 to 15 percent and increases new mitochondria growth after four days, thus increasing stem cells! So fast away, but consult your practitioner first.
- Most people eat a glycemic index of 80 or more. Stay below 50.
- Low GI diets give you time-released energy.
- Low GI keeps you in the fat-burning zone.

* Shari Leiberman, *Glycemic Index*, A4M 14th International Congress on Anti-Aging Medicine, conference lecture notes, September 2006.

- Low GI diets decrease C-reactive protein (CRP), fix insulin resistance, and do not lower BMR.*

Of course, your actual success in developing an anti-inflammatory eating pattern depends on knowing exactly what foods to consume and which ones not to. To help you plan your intake, Appendix 1 in this book provides a detailed list of anti-inflammatory foods you can seek out when doing your grocery shopping. You'll also find guidance on how much you need of omega-3, -6, -7, and -9 oils and other key components of your anti-inflammatory lifestyle.

I recommend incorporating the low-glycemic foods listed in Appendix 1 when grocery shopping. Since so many items in the grocery store are not conducive to a healthy life, you'll need to go well-armed with information to guide you to the right choices. And, perhaps not surprisingly, many of the right choices are different than what we've been told are "right." We'll talk about some of those in the next chapter.

BIBLICAL NUTRITION

The Lord has provided all the foods we need for a healthy body. He gave us the perfect plan.

The Mediterranean diet consists of a lot of these foods. Unfortunately, we have processed the nutritional value out of many of the foods that were created to preserve shelf life.

Important key things to remember are: The Almighty created three main categories of unclean classes of creatures that are scavengers, acting as garbage disposals, to clean up toxins and dead carcasses from the earth, air, and sea. The Holy Bible gives the descriptions and instructions of the clean and unclean animals in Leviticus.

1. **Certain animal species of the earth**. These include the swine or pig. Other creatures we are told not to eat are from the cat family, the camel, rabbits, fox, kangaroo, horses, and dogs.
2. **Birds of the air and winged insects**. These include the eagle, the vulture, the buzzard, the falcon, and ravens. There are certain insects that are okay to eat, but I think I'd rather fast.
3. **Living things of the waters**. Many sea creatures (seafood) are "bottom dwellers," which were created to clean the bottoms of the oceans, lakes, and rivers. If they don't have scales, do not eat them.

There is a correct way an animal (cattle, chicken, lambs, for example) is killed or slaughtered. Meat from an animal that has been stressed when slaughtered in an

* Leiberman, *Glycemic Index.*

inhumane manner has a high pH that affects the color, flavor, and texture of the meat.

Kosher meats are slaughtered in such a way that unconsciousness is instantaneous and death occurs almost immediately. This has the opposite effect on the meat of the animal.

Some cheeses may include pork rind in the processing. If there is a symbol for kosher on the packaging, it is free of any of these products, and is meant to indicate that the animals were humanely slaughtered. This may not be the case, so do your own homework. There are numerous kosher symbols.

Listed below are the clean foods found throughout the Bible. I strongly recommend you follow the clean vs. unclean biblical instructions, as they were given to protect your health. Always choose organic, non-GMO, and non-bioengineered products. It's important to always read the labels, especially the small print.[*,†]

1. Almonds
2. Anise
3. Barley
4. Beans
5. Bitter herbs
6. Cheese
7. Ceylon cinnamon
8. Cucumbers
9. Cumin
10. Figs
11. Fish with scales
12. Flax
13. Fruits
14. Garlic
15. Grains
16. Grapes
17. Grass-fed whole milk
18. Herbs
19. Honey
20. Hyssop
21. Leeks
22. Legumes
23. Lentils

---

* Cecelia Marie Desonia, *God-Given Food: A Bible Study and Beyond . . .* (CreateSpace Independent Publishing Platform, June 22, 2017).

† Reginald Cherry, MD, *The Bible Cure* (Siloam; First edition, 1998).

24. Millet
25. Mint
26. Mustard seeds
27. Nuts
28. Olives and olive oil
29. Onions
30. Pistachio nuts
31. Pomegranates
32. Seeds
33. Spelt
34. Sprouts
35. Vinegar
36. Wheat

Important naturopathic things to remember:

- Eat only fruits and vegetables that are in season.
- Too much heat and overcooking destroy enzymes and some vitamins.
- Eat a variety of whole grains (soak them first to reduce the phytic-acid content).
- Eat a variety of seeds and nuts (soak these also).
- Season foods with sprouts, herbs, and spices.
- Use extra-virgin olive oil in cooking and salads.
- Use dried fruits for desserts (i.e., raisins, dates, and figs).
- Eat small portions of meat the size of your palm.
- Avoid chemical additives.

CHAPTER 8

The Good, the Bad, and the Beneficial

Misinformation has clouded our thinking about many of the items we consume every day. And even if the misinformation was well-intended (which it is at times), it is still misinformation that can deprive you of nutritional advantages of healthy eating. We'll look at several mis-informational myths that you're no doubt well-acquainted with.

- MYTH: Unpasteurized milk is dangerous. The truth is skim milk is a toxic by-product from the dairy industry.
- MYTH: Salt is bad for you. While refined salt is bad for you, unprocessed salt is good for your health and your heart.
- MYTH: Fluoride is good for you. The truth is that a study in *Environmental Health* has deemed fluoride a neuro-excitotoxin.*

The Benefits of Raw Milk

Today's commercial milk producing cows are bred to produce large amounts of milk. And the process of "pushing" cows to overproduce results in milk that contains high levels of growth hormones. These cows are fed mostly genetically-modified grains, and they produce three times more milk than old-fashioned cows.

As a result, they live only about forty-two months compared to about twelve years for grass-fed cows. All of this industrial-strength milk production pushes them to their "udder limits." Simply put, they wear out. And guess what that means for the milk you drink from them? It produces all kinds of nasty health issues.†

* International Academy of Oral Medicine and Toxicology (IAOMT), Fluoride Facts: Sources, Exposure and Health Effects, https://iaomt.org/resources/fluoride-facts/.

† PPNF (Price-Pottenger Nutrition Foundation), Journal of Health and Healing, https://price-pottenger.org/.

In 2002, Weston A. Price warned us about this:*

> "During the heating process, the aforementioned sulphydryl compounds impart a very strong cabbagy off-flavor to UHT milk that is most noticeable immediately after heating. These compounds dissipate during storage, but approximately one month into storage, UHT milk begins to deteriorate and is described in the industry as "stale." In the later stages of storage, a bitter taste develops and then it undergoes "age gelation," a process in which the milk becomes more viscous and eventually loses fluidity. So, it seems the optimum time to drink UHT milk with any degree of enjoyment, if that's even possible, is limited to the interval between the dissipation of the cabbage flavor and the onset of staleness, bitterness and gelatinous conditions. In the United States, these off-flavors seem to go unnoticed, which makes me wonder whether some kind of flavorings or other chemicals are being added to UHT milk? If the whole industry does this, they don't need to list such additives on the label because it is an "industry standard."

More recently, Sally Fallon, founder and president of the Weston A. Price Foundation, noted that "the *intrinsic properties of* milk, including its pH and nutrient content, make it an excellent medium for the survival and growth of pathogenic bacteria, applies only to pasteurized milk, not raw milk."†

Homogenized milk has also been linked to heart disease, and worst of all, consumers have been duped into believing that low-fat and skim-milk products are good for them. The truth is, though, that only by marketing low-fat and skim milk as health foods can the modern dairy industry get rid of the excess poor-quality reduced-fat milk from modern high-production herds. This is toxic waste meant for your consumption. Raw milk, by contrast, is very beneficial to your health in almost every way that pasteurized milk is not. Here's an overview of what raw milk offers, most of which is destroyed in the pasteurization process:

- **Lactoperoxidase**—An enzyme that seeks out and destroys bad bacteria. It is found in all mammals' secretions such as breast milk, tears, and saliva.
- **Lactoferrin—**This enzyme takes away iron from pathogenic bacteria and stimulates the immune system. It ensures complete assimilation of iron by infants.
- **Polysaccharides**—These protect the gut wall and encourage the growth of good bacteria in the gastrointestinal (GI) tract.
- **Bioactive milk peptides**—These help to combat insomnia.

---

* WAPF, Ultra-Pasteurized Milk, 2002, http://www.westonaprice.org/health-topics/modern-foods/ultra-pasteurized-milk/#gsc.tab=0.

† *WAPF Journal* (Fall 2015), 243–45.

- **Medium chain triglycerides (MCTs)**—A very favorable type of fat that disrupts cellular walls in pathogenic bacteria. MCTs are also found in coconut milk.
- **Enzymes**—To disrupt bacterial cell walls.
- **Antibodies**—Their purpose is to bind foreign microbes to prevent them from migrating outside the gut. This prevents leaky gut syndrome (LGS).
- **White blood cells (WBCs)**—These white blood cells produce antibodies against specific bacteria and are especially critical for infants.
- **B-lymphocytes**—Cells that kill foreign microbes and send out messages to other parts of the immune system.
- **Macrophages**—Components that engulf foreign proteins in bacteria. These mop up unwanted proteins that can cause autoimmunity.
- **Neutrophils**—These immune cells mobilize some components of the immune system.
- **T-lymphocytes**—These immune cells produce immune-strengthening compounds and multiply when harmful bacteria are present.
- **Lysozymes**—These compounds digest bacterial cell walls.
- **Hormones and growth factors**—Stimulate the maturation of colonocytes, thereby preventing leaky gut syndrome (LGS).
- **Mucins**—These proteins stick to harmful bacteria and viruses, thereby preventing them from attaching to the mucosal wall and causing disease. A very useful substance in restoring gut wall integrity.
- **Oligosaccharides**—Special sugars to protect important compounds from being destroyed by stomach acid and enzymes. These also bind to bacteria and prevent them from sticking to the gut lining.
- **Vitamin B12-binding protein**—This protein reduces the levels of vitamin B12 in the gut by binding to B12. This renders B12 inactive to harmful bacteria which need it for growth. This protein also ensures complete assimilation of B12 by the infant.
- **Bifidus factor**—A complex of beneficial bacteria that promotes the growth of *Lactobacillum bifidus*, a helpful bacterial component in the baby's gut which helps crowd out pathogenic bacteria.
- **Glycosphingolipids**—These prevent intestinal distress.
- **Conjugated linoleic acid (CLA)**—An essential fatty acid with strong anticancer properties.
- **Fibronectin**—This helps to repair damaged tissue in the gut by increasing the antimicrobial activity of macrophages.

On the other hand, pasteurization is actually linked to a variety of problems: Colic in infants, arthritis, heart disease, osteoporosis, and behavioral problems in children. Pasteurization was instituted in the 1920s to combat TB, infant diarrhea, undulant fever, and other diseases caused by poor animal nutrition and dirty production methods. At the time, infected water supplies were also a problem. But times have changed and effective water treatment, stainless steel tanks, milking machines, refrigerated trucks, and improved testing methods make pasteurization absolutely unnecessary for public protection.*

It's noteworthy that powdered skim milk, a source of dangerous oxidized cholesterol and neurotoxic amino acids, is added to 1 percent and 2 percent milk. Because it is left over after the removal of cream, skim milk is essentially a waste by-product of the dairy industry.

Regarding other commonly used dairy products, the Weston A. Price Foundation notes:

- No one should use skim milk, margarine, or canola oil—*ever*! (I strongly agree.)
- Low-fat yogurts and sour cream contain *muco-polysaccharide slime* solely to give them body. Yummy! Stay far away from 98 percent of all yogurt. If it's pasteurized, put it back on the shelf.
- Remember: Low-fat means high sugar!
- Pale butter from hay-fed cows contains colorings to imitate the vitamin-rich butter from grass-fed cows. Use grass-fed butter only (such as Kerrygold).
- Bioengineered enzymes are used in large-scale cheese production.

So, there's plenty you've been led to believe about milk that's wrong. Stop allowing yourself to be spoon-fed by the dairy industry and the GMO food mega-giants. Ask the crazy crunchy moms. They aren't so crazy after all.

Iodine and Its Importance

Iodine is one of the most important nutrients required by the human body. It is essential to the proper alkalization of your cells.† This mineral also contributes to cognitive development in children. Adequate levels of iodine have been shown to prevent cancer and are antiviral, antibacterial, and antifungal.‡

Yet the US consumption of iodine is incredibly deficient. According to Jorge Flechas, MD,§ a world authority on iodine, most people have iodine levels that are virtually undetectable.

How have we come to be so lacking in this critical component of good health? A wide variety of causes are in play:

---

* Raw Milk Institute, Nutritional Benefits of Raw Milk, https://www.rawmilkinstitute.org/about-raw-milk/#nutrition

† IAOMT, conference lecture notes, 2018.

‡ David Brownstein, MD, *Iodine: Why You Need It* (Medical Alternative Press, 2014).

§ Jorge Flechas, MD, *Iodine Deficiency and Its Treatment*, https://www.youtube.com/watch?v=ooHypvctEp4.

- Nationwide, the soil, and hence the crops grown in it, is depleted of iodine.
- Diets without ocean fish or sea vegetables such as seaweed are devoid of iodine.
- Inadequate use of iodized salt (from low-salt diets). Your thyroid gland enlarges to capture more iodine (goiter). Iodized salt contains only a minute amount anyway, the rest being sodium.
- Diets high in pastas and breads which contain bromide inhibit the body's absorption of iodine.
- Bromide binds to the iodine receptors and displaces iodine. Tell your dentist.
- Chloride has the same effect as bromide, plus it kills lactobacillus in the gut. Don't drink tap water.
- Fluoride (such as that in treated municipal water and at your local dentistry office) also contributes to the inhibition of iodine binding.
- Tell your dental hygienist not to clean your children's teeth (or yours) with prophy paste that contains fluoride.
- Vegan and vegetarian diets are lacking in iodine.
- Sucralose (contains chlorinated table sugar) displaces iodine.
- Medications (especially inhalers and SSRIs—selective serotonin reuptake inhibitors).
- Any meds that have fluoro- as a prefix.
- Aging.

It is estimated that 95 percent of the population in the United States is deficient in iodine intake. According to Guy Abraham, dosing of iodine at 50–100 mg per day may be necessary to reduce the oxidative DNA damage caused by an iodine deficiency. The "official" (low) recommended daily doses of iodine are ineffective against cancer development and actually make existing cancers more aggressive.

Low levels also cause the size of breast tumors to increase. On the other hand, adequate levels of iodine can treat conditions such as fibrocystic breast disease, Dupuytren's contracture (a progressive deformity of the hand), polycystic ovary syndrome, autoimmune diseases, excess mucus production, fatigue, hemorrhoids, periodontal disease, headaches (including migraines), keloids, ovarian cysts, parotid duct stones, Peyronie's disease (fibrous scar tissue in the penis), sebaceous cysts, and thyroid disorders.*

Without adequate iodine levels, you cannot achieve the proper cellular membrane voltage of -20mv that I explained in chapter 1—an absolute necessity to maintain cellular healing. Iodine deficiency is responsible for our high rates of

* Scott Laird, ND and Jodi Laird; Laird Wellness; Thyroid Issues, https://rumble.com/v36jefp-thyroid-issues.html.

cancer—especially breast, lung, prostate, and ovarian cancers. Iodine also functions as a strong antioxidant.*, †

With regard to breast cancer, in particular, iodine modulates estrogenic receptors in the breasts and inhibits the spread of cancer cells and as a result, inhibits tumor formation. So, take 12.5 to 50 milligrams per day according to Dr. David Brownstein, Jorge Flechas, and Dr. Guy Abraham, world leaders in iodine research. They also suggest you must salt away with unrefined salt. Tell that to your cardiologist.

The Acidic-Alkaline Shift

Another underestimated necessity of good health is the maintenance of the proper balance of acidity and alkalinity in your 70 to 100 trillion cells, as measured by the pH of your blood. (I'd still like to know who's counting all those cells.) This is extremely problematic, because most all disease states—including both acute and chronic conditions—thrive in acidic environments. That means, if your body is acidic (low in pH), you are more prone to disease. Acidic regions of your body facilitate problems because they decrease oxygen availability and attract immune modulators and anaerobic bugs, yeast and the like. However, stomach acidity needs to be increased. Please note that various parts of the body operate at different pH levels.

Infection and disease states will cause plasma shifts in the blood and localized "acidic regions" in the body. **Here's a list of specific diseases that can be triggered by poor pH balance and acidosis (high acidity):**

The top three world-wide conditions (as per the *American Dental Association Journal*, stated in many monthly articles)‡:

- Gingivitis
- Periodontal disease
- Dental decay

as well as:

- Crohn's disease
- Colitis
- Osteoarthritis
- Atherosclerosis
- Cancerous areas
- Autoimmune diseases
- Bone spurs, due to acid imbalance needed for bone building
- Chronic fatigue, due in part to poor muscle and cognitive function.

---

* Brownstein, *Iodine: Why You Need It*.

† TTAC, Conference Series, 2017, 2019, 2021, https://thetruthaboutcancer.com/category/videos/.

‡ ADA, et al., http://www.ada.org/search-results#q=Decay&sort=relevancy.

This is why the homeostatic control between acidity and alkalinity is such a big deal. So, to help you manage your grocery shopping with proper alkalinity in mind, I've included a list of pH-friendly foods in Appendix 2. Again, it's 80 percent alkaline foods. Remember, alkaline foods donate electrons to the system.

If you want to manage your pH balance, what do you do?

Here's a checklist of ways you can create a lifestyle conducive to healthy pH levels:

1. Eat alkaline-friendly foods (see Appendix 2).
2. Drink alkaline water, but remember to add back the minerals.
3. Control your stress levels by increasing your parasympathetic nervous system (PSNS) through proper breathing techniques.
4. Decrease the sympathetic nervous system response (reactive stress, et al.). Save the stress for when it is truly stressful.
5. Increase mineral balance and control aldosterone (a hormone that manages salt and water in the body, resulting in proper blood pressure management).
6. Increase metabolism by increasing oxygen consumption (proper sleep and increase nitric oxide (NO). This is what ozone does.
7. Sleep at least 7 hours per night. If you can't, seek help.

Of these items, perhaps the single most important factor is stress control. When you increase stress, you increase the sympathetic nervous system response, which decreases oxygen consumption. This increase in stress then increases cortisol levels and increases the cellular metabolic waste of the cell. This in turn, increases cortisol in a process known as pregnenolone steal that occurs in the glucocorticoid pathway of your adrenal glands.*

Stress also affects the CO_2 and oxygen exchange system by lowering oxygen levels needed for complete oxidation to occur. Incomplete oxidation ("metabolic exhaust") causes an increase in free radicals, and this greatly reduces ATP formation in the mitochondria.

In general, diseased cells are created by acidic changes in pH, a decrease in voltage, and lowered oxygen. When cells are deficient in oxygen, spirochetes (destructive bacteria) crawl out of the red blood cells and are set loose in the body.†

How do you know if you're out of balance in the pH department? Fortunately, that's not very difficult to find out. It's actually fairly easy to test your pH balance

* Kurt Woeller, DO, *Resolving Chronic Stress Disorders,* 6-DVD-set module course, https://toxicitymasterycourse.com/.

† Dr. David Kennedy, IAOMT conference lecture notes, San Diego, 2014.

on your own. You can get pH test strips at a health-food store or your local pharmacy, and they're inexpensive—about $10 for a roll.

When exposed to urine, the strip turns color, which you then compare to the chart you get with the strips. Each color is assigned a number representing your pH level. I recommend that people test their first morning urine for seven days in a row to determine their average pH, and even better, test before dinner as well. Testing twice a day should really nail down the results.

If the average of your seven-day urinary pH levels is between 6.6 and 7, that's good. Keep in mind that stress can make you acidic, as can *all* medications, toxins (such as mercury and lead), and intestinal infections (including yeast and parasites).

If your readings are too acidic, increase your intake of fruits, vegetables, and minerals, until your average pH value is between 6.6 and 7. Also change your breathing pattern. It will help to add alkaline water to your daily regimen. However, if you change your diet but see no improvement, other factors may be involved, and you should consult with your healthcare professional. If you discover that your pH is out of balance, there are specific steps you can take to bring your body back to its optimal alkaline state—a condition known as homeostasis. The endocannabinoid system regulates the homeostasis of your body. I've outlined below some very doable steps you can take to balance your pH level. Balance your oral pH, keeping it no lower than 6.6 (7.0 is even better). See Soda Doping below for guidance on how to do this.

1. Increase your stomach acid by taking Hydrozyme from Biotics Research Corp.
2. Take iodine, 12.5 to 25 mg. Iodoral is a good choice (tableted Lugol's solution or Pro-thera-iodine complex). Balance with selenium, 800 mcg. (Get your levels tested.)
3. Alkalinize your water with ozone, distilled, reverse osmosis, Kangen, or a Berkey water filter.*
4. Take probiotics every day. (A good source is Ancient Nutrition.†)
5. Eat lots of vegetables and alkaline fruits (preferably ripe and in season).
6. Pearl Silica Drops®, five to ten drops per day (to bowel tolerance). Children take three to five drops per day. Trace Mineral Drops by ConcenTrace® Mineral Drops. About ½ tsp a day.
7. Reduce your stress.
8. Reduce your calorie intake (CR—caloric restriction). In other words, eat less.

---

* Scott Laird, ND and Jodi Laird; Laird Wellness, How to Make Immune Boosting Water, https://rumble.com/v4cd2i0-how-to-make-immune-boosting-water.html.

† Ancient Nutrition, https://ancientnutrition.com/pages/probiotics-digestionAncientNutrition.com.

9. Limit or eliminate medications. All of your meds are acidic. (Work with your doctor on this one.)
10. Detoxify using the Detoxification Protocol.*
11. Maintain proper oxidation in your body through limited exercise and increased nitric oxide. This increases the microvasculature. I recommend the best, Cardio Miracle.†
12. Eliminate mercury fillings—but only the correct way. See a biological dentist.

I mentioned Soda Doping which is a home remedy for improving your pH balance quickly. It both alkalinizes your body and improves your day-to-day endurance. The process is simple: Put a teaspoon of baking soda in water (make sure it's aluminum-free); swish it in your mouth; brush your teeth; then rinse with the soda solution.

Here is what it does for you:

1. Decreases heartburn (if hyperacidity is the problem—which it usually is *not*).
2. Alkalinizes your oral mucosa (a good thing).
3. Helps with exercise stamina.
4. Helps neutralize alcohol and boosts NO.
5. Takes lactic acid out of your system (good for your muscles).

So, raw milk, iodine, and proper pH balance. What's the next common nutrient we need but haven't been told the truth about or have been lied to concerning its use?

The Assault on Salt

Everybody knows salt is bad for you. It causes high blood pressure and all sorts of associated problems. Right? Unfortunately, everybody does seem to know that, and once again, we're dealing with a serious case of misinformation. Salt is actually extremely good for you, but it has to be the right kind of salt.

Although we "moderns" demonize salt, historically speaking, we're in a small minority of people who have so badly misunderstood the value of this wonderful creation. A quick review of how people have valued salt reveals a tremendous gap between what they knew and what we think we know. Here are a few historical salt facts for you:

* http://www.drlokensgard.com/shop.

† Cardio Miracle, *The Cardio Miracle Story*, https://cardiomiracle.com/pages/the-cardio-miracle-story.

- In 450 BC, Hippocrates recognized the healing power of salt.
- Roman soldiers were paid in salt.
- Salt was an expensive, highly sought-after commodity.
- The word *salary* comes from the word *salaria*, which comes from the word *salt.*
- Salt was used for preservation, storage, and transport.
- Salt was considered a divine substance by Yehovah—we are the salt of the earth.
- The Celtic word for salt also means sacred or holy.

So, where do our imagined problems with salt come from? They stem from the reality that most commercially purchased table salts these days are refined or processed in such a way that it turns on us. Not only are all of the key nutrient minerals refined *out*, but the mineral imbalances left *in* cause serious problems. Processing causes an imbalance in mineral ratios, and as a result, it becomes mostly sodium chloride—bad for you. This alone can drive up blood pressure.[*]

On the other hand, *unrefined* salt, also known as Celtic Sea salt, Redmond Sea Salt, and Himalayan pink salt, is extremely good for you. These salts contain as many as 80 macro- as well as micro-minerals—and in the correct balance.

We have been done a major disservice by the food industry with regard to necessary salt requirements. Salt is needed in our bodies as cofactors in thousands of different enzymatic reactions occurring every second. It's also required to maintain proper cellular membrane voltage. (Does the significance of voltage sound familiar yet?) This in turn, allows for proper ion channel function and voltage at the cellular membrane, which determines proper active and passive cellular membrane transport.[†]

Mineral salt also helps in the process of teeth and bone remineralization. Here are a few facts about salt:

- The USDA recommends that you reduce your salt intake to 3.5 grams per day.
- You actually need 7 grams of unrefined salt every day to increase electrolytic balance. Processed salt contains anticaking compounds: ferrocyanide, fluoride, and synthetic aluminosilicate, and *none* of these compounds are good for you, but for some reason, the USDA and the FDA have decided that you need these ingredients.
- Processed salt contains only sodium and chloride with a miniscule amount of iodine added to prevent goiter.

---

* David Brownstein, MD and Sheryl Shenefelt, CN, *The Guide to Healthy Eating*, (Center for Holistic Medicine, 2010) 99–106.

† Allergy Research Group, Focus Newsletter, http://www.allergyresearchgroup.com/education.

- Sodium activates glial cells, thereby activating sodium ion channels, but you need other minerals in order to balance out the sodium. This, in part, is what makes refined salt not so healthy.*

The bottom line is that salt is an essential nutrient. What does essential mean? It contains required minerals your body does not have the capability to make on its own. Therefore, you must consume them every day to get what you need. The same is true with EFAs and amino acids (however, not all amino acids are essential). If you don't consume these on a daily basis, your cells cannot heal properly, due to the lowered voltage, and chronic pain and disease can be the result.

Himalayan pink salt is mined in Nepal and is the very best salt for you. Healthful, unrefined salt taken on a daily basis can have many of the health benefits noted below.

1. Unrefined salt increases metabolism and can decrease dental decay.
2. Increases voltage and normalizes your heart rhythm.
3. Increases adrenal function.
4. Salt that is *refined* can lower your pH level and raise your blood pressure.
5. Water and salt are necessary for detoxification, metabolism, and transport of nutrients, as well as optimal functioning of the hormonal, nervous, and immune systems.
6. When you crave salt, it's usually due to decreased adrenal function.
7. Minerals are alkalinizing.
8. The mineral Mg+ is a cofactor in over four hundred reactions.
9. Minerals are buffering agents that reduce acidity and balance your blood pH level.
10. Without the balancing of trace minerals, processed salt provides too much sodium and throws the electrolytic balance into chaos. The consequences of this are: mineral deficiencies, increased acidity, and the onset of chronic degenerative disease (cancer and aging).
11. Almost all Americans are deficient in minerals—especially iodine, magnesium, zinc, and selenium.†, ‡
12. Most people are also potassium deficient (potassium maintains fluid balance and stimulates muscle contraction). When potassium levels are normal, blood pressure and fluid levels are maintained at optimal balance.§

---

* Ibid.

† Life Extension, *The Science of a Healthier Life*, Journal Articles (Collectors Edition, Feb 2011), 49.

‡ Life Extension, *The Science of a Healthier Life*, Journal Articles (October 2009).

§ Dr. John LaPuma, *The Power of Potassium for Nerve and Muscle Function,* http://www.drjohnlapuma.com/wellness-and-health/the-power-of-potassium-for-muscle-and-nerve-function/.

13. Kidney patients should monitor their processed salt intake because salt is excreted by the kidneys. If you are in renal failure or have a decreased ability to eliminate salt, you must be careful. If you have any questions, talk to your healthcare provider; make sure they are trained by the A4M or the IFM.
14. Low-salt diets have been shown to raise fasting insulin levels. (This makes and keeps the fat on you.)
15. Magnesium is a muscle-relaxing mineral but must be balanced with calcium—the right kind of calcium—calcium citrate or malate.
16. Magnesium and potassium have a direct antihypertensive effect.
17. Potassium deficiencies have been shown to cause elevated blood pressure in many studies.*
18. Refined salt should *never* be consumed—just like margarine, skim or low-fat milk, or low-fat anything. But you should consume at least 3 to 7 grams of unrefined and unprocessed salt per day (the equivalent of 1.5 to 2 teaspoons of salt per day).

So now you have the permission and motivation you need: Salt away, raise your voltage, and increase your adrenal function. Get away from the false notions we've been led to believe about what we eat and how to stay healthy—not the least of which is the never-ending concern so many of us have about our weight. It's the health issue that has more people preoccupied than any other.

The problem is, too few "experts" are giving us the right answers (and corresponding solutions) to the huge question: Why are we fat? We are fat because we consume low-fat, trans fat, plastic-fat diets that are high in fake sugar, low in nutrient value, causing insulin levels that are out of control; we are all stressed out; our hormones are all out of whack, and that's what is making us fat and our kids fat and giving all of us too many heart attacks.

If you don't believe me, just go people watching at any major mall, airport, or grocery store in America. The result of our *burgeoning population* ends up as toxicity! So, let's dive into this major "American phenomenon."

---

* Life Extension, *The Science of a Healthier Life, Slash Inches off Your Waistline,* Journal Article (May 2022).

CHAPTER 9

It's a Toxic World

On the night before George Washington died, the president's doctors administered a concoction of calomel (mercurous chloride) and did a bloodletting procedure during which 35 to 40 percent of his blood was removed from his body. Our first president, who had been managing his plantation from horseback in apparently good health only forty-eight hours before, died the next day.*

You might be tempted to think we've come a long way since 1799, and if so, you'd be right . . . in some ways. Certainly, we know not to "bleed" a patient or infuse a sick person's body with mercury (or do we?). And the results of modern medical procedures in saving trauma patients borders on the miraculous. But with regard to nutrition and whole-body health, in some respects, we are living in a world of falsified science.

Modern nutritional and medical practices often are not much better than injecting a poison like mercury into our veins or our teeth. And the problem of internal toxicity is complicated by the plethora of toxicity in our environment these days.

Toxins All Around

Some people face an acutely toxic environment in the workplace, but most of us don't work in chemical plants, mines, or industrial waste sites. The rest of us, though, endure toxins in the environment that are virtually unavoidable, especially in our homes. Yet we don't have to succumb to the potentially lethal effects. There are steps you can take to live as toxin-free as possible, but as with most everything associated with truly healthful living (THL), fighting back first requires getting educated on what challenges we face.

The "big three" non-work-related toxic situations we face are food and beverages, air and water, and personal products. Let's look at each of these.

---

* Dr. Thomas Lokensgard, *Medicine and Treatment During the American Revolution*, Old Glory DAR Chapter (Franklin, TN, Program Lecture, July 2011).

Food and Beverages

The challenge we confront as to what we consume begins externally because we have a choice of what to put in our mouths. External influences may tempt us to make bad choices. Consider, for instance, the implication of a few startling facts about what we consume if we do not limit our consumption of processed foods:

In America, the average per capita consumption of chemical food additives is about ten pounds per year.*

That means, your liver has to filter the equivalent of a one-hundred-pound barrel of foreign substances every ten years.

Even the healthiest individuals are undermined by this toxic load.

Our Creator has designed each cell in your body (except RBCs) to be capable of fixing themselves through the detoxification and repair process. But when the system becomes overloaded with ambient or internal toxins, it breaks down. Clearly, our choices about what to eat are critical to good health.

Air and Water

It's been estimated that something like 650 different industrial chemicals have been released into our air and water each year. This amounts to about 7.1 billion pounds of toxic agents.†

Personal Products

We've come to accept a false sense of security in our grocery stores and think that whatever "they" sell us must be "safe" or "it wouldn't be allowed." Remember: The FDA protects "them," not you. As a result, most of us are exposed to toxic chemicals every day without giving it a second thought, as we use shampoo, deodorant, mouthwash, hair spray, body lotions, cosmetics, toothpaste, and detergents. It must be okay, right?

If you read the labels on many of these common products, you'll be astounded to discover the waste-dump of ingredients. Consider these examples:

- My very favorite is propylene glycol, also known as antifreeze—in many food and cosmetic products. This is why you must start reading labels.
- Toothpaste often contains sugars, carrageenan, sodium fluoride, D&C yellow #10, FD&C blue #1, flavor, non-plant-based glycerin, sodium lauryl sulfate, sodium saccharin, sorbitol, titanium dioxide, trisodium phosphate, water, and xanthan gum. In deodorant, you'll find aluminum chlorohydrate, butylated hydroxytoluene (BHT), fragrance, PPG-11

---

* IAOMT, Conference lecture notes, 2018.

† *Daily Hampshire Gazette*; "Rain Yields High Levels of Mercury" (September 19, 2000). http://www.gazettenet.com/.

stearyl ether or PPG-15, steareth-2, steareth-20, water, D&C yellow #10, and FD&C red #4.

The Toxic Results

There is no way to completely escape this sea of chemicals we live in, and sadly, years of exposure can result in a number of chronic conditions. These include:

- Chronic fatigue syndrome
- Environmental sensitivities imbalance (also called MCS—multiple chemical sensitivities)
- Candida overgrowth
- Chronic pain and inflammation
- Allergies and thyroid issues
- Degenerative joint disease (DJD) and arthralgia (inflammatory joint pain)
- Hormonal problems
- Intestinal distress
- Cognitive dysfunction*

In a recent study led by Mount Sinai School of Medicine in New York,† researchers found after testing for 210 toxic chemicals, the average test subject had ninety-one industrial compounds, pollutants, and other chemicals in their blood and urine. The nine subjects carried an average toxic burden of:

- Fifty-three chemicals linked to cancer
- Sixty-two chemicals that are toxic to the brain and nervous system
- Fifty-eight chemicals that interfere with the hormone system
- Fifty-five chemicals associated with birth defects or abnormal development
- Fifty-five chemicals toxic to the reproductive system
- Fifty-three chemicals toxic to the immune system

But that's not all. The laboratory also found forty-eight different PCBs in the nine subjects even though PCBs were banned in the United States over twenty-five years ago. It's evident that no matter how diligent we are with a clean diet, we cannot escape the toxins in our environment. The chronically ill may be suffering from a toxic load that they cannot overcome, but as we continue to learn,

---

* Roger Deutsch and Rudy Rivera, MD, *Your Hidden Food Allergies Are Making You Fat* (Prima Lifestyles, 2002), 152–55.

† Forbes, Industrial Chemicals Lurking in Your Bloodstream, https://www.forbes.com/2010/01/21/toxic-chemicals-bpa-lifestyle-health-endocrine-disruptors.html.

Toxic-Free Future, Persistent, Bioaccumulative, and Toxic Chemicals, https://toxicfreefuture.org/toxic-chemicals/persistent-bioaccumulative-and-toxic-chemicals-pbts/.

by building our own immunities and guarding ourselves in ways we can control, there's a lot we can do to minimize the effect of the external environment. One particular, nearly ubiquitous, environmental toxin deserves particular attention.

Is Fluoride Safe—or Even Effective?

Fluoride, a halogen on the periodic chemistry chart, is toxic even at very low levels and can be deadly in children at higher levels. This chemical compound exists everywhere in nature and has a few beneficial effects, but most of what it does is negative for your health.*

There are conflicting views and conclusions about fluoride, based on a wide array of special interests, vested money, and, in my opinion, some very flawed studies. But I'm not the only one who questions whether fluoride is good for us. The prestigious British medical journal *The Lancet* has now officially labeled fluoride as a neuro-excitotoxin. Such substances are known to cause the range of problems outlined below.

- Cancer (especially osteosarcomas).
- Mottling of tooth enamel. These are white or brown spots on the teeth; the condition is also called fluorosis.
- Osteoporosis and bone cancer in horses and other animals.†
- Death in children who have swallowed or eaten large amounts of toothpaste containing fluoride.
- Birth defects at higher levels.
- Brittle or hardened tooth enamel that cracks (similar to the bisphosphonates—in the form of drugs of the past, like Boniva).
- Hypothyroidism, by interfering with iodine (also on the periodic chart), replacing it on the tyrosine ring, and thus diminishing production of T3, the active form of your thyroid hormone.‡
- Bone tumors upon fluoride exposure, causing increased bone turnover and altered mineral metabolism. (Note: a very small amount of fluoride is necessary for bone formation. In a study of the workplace, chronic fluoride exposure resulted in immune depression in all workers.§

Fluoride has also been shown to cause negative effects on numerous organ systems including:

- The kidneys

---

* IAOMT, Fluoride Facts, https://iaomt.org/resources/fluoride-facts/fluoride-exposure-human-health-risks/.

† IAOMT, Fluoride Resources, https://iaomt.org/resources/.

‡ Brownstein, *Iodine: Why You Need It.*

§ Roger Deutsch and Rudy Rivera, MD, *Your Hidden Food Allergies Are Making You Fat* (Prima Lifestyles, 2002) 152–55.

- The reproductive system
- The cardiovascular system
- The brain
- The neurological system
- The liver
- The pineal gland
- The breasts and glandular system
- The immune function and thyroid function

And guess what? Even though the most-cited reason for using fluoride is dental health, fluoride tablets and drops have both been shown to be ineffective in reducing tooth decay. According to the International Association of Oral Medicine and Toxicology (IAOMT), fluoride products have still not yet been proven as safe or effective. They have, however, been shown to cause skin eruptions, gastric distress, headaches, and weakness, which disappear when fluoride use is discontinued.*

Systemic exposure to fluoride during tooth development causes dental fluorosis, which is a permanent disfigurement, causing mottling of the enamel. This negatively affects bone metabolism and the calcification process. Lifelong exposure even to low levels of fluoride will increase the likelihood of hip fractures. What's more, fluoride has been shown to increase the frequency of cancers at the epiphysial growth plates, the part of your bones where growth occurs.†

Fluoride is a "bully" chemical in that it pushes all of its halide cousins out of the way and displaces iodine in the thyroid tyrosine ring; as such, it is listed as one of the ten most common household toxins. And the effect of fluoride is cumulative. Its presence builds up over time, primarily in bones. During their growth years, children accumulate fluoride more rapidly in their bones than adults do. Chronic ingestion of 1 ppm daily of fluoride gradually accumulates in critical sites, and over decades will negatively impact bone health and increase the potential for hip fractures.

The fluoride in your toothpaste is a pharmaceutical-grade sodium fluoride, stannous fluoride or sodium mono-fluoro-phosphate, but it does little in the way of increasing the strength of your teeth. The fluoride in municipal water supplies is a silicofluoride, a highly contaminated, hazardous-waste by-product of the phosphate fertilizer industry. The EPA does not even allow this toxic by-product to be put into landfills or be discarded into rivers or oceans. So why is it fit for you and your family's consumption, especially your children and grandchildren? It isn't.

---

* IAOMT, Fluoride, https://iaomt.org/resources/position-papers/iaomt-fluoride-position-paper/.

† International Society for Fluoride Research, Budapest Study, 21st Congress Budapest, Hungary.

Here is a personal experience I had when I was attending the University of Minnesota School of Dentistry my freshman year. I was working on a biochemistry laboratory project with a world-class PhD named Leon Singer. We were measuring fluoride ion migration across the enamel by a process called iontophoresis. The project took nine weeks, or one school quarter, as we diligently painted a substance on extracted teeth called Duraphat. This substance contained lots of fluoride. At the end of the school quarter, we measured the fluoride ion migration across the enamel and found it to be negligible. So, the next time your dentist wants to bill you or your insurance company for a one-minute fluoride treatment, share this with them!

All of the recent large-scale studies on the relationship between drinking water, fluoridation, and tooth decay show that fluoridation does not reduce tooth decay. It makes the enamel matrix more brittle, thus more subject to fracture.

What's more, children's health appears to be better in non-fluoridated areas. Fluoridation has also been reported to delay eruption of the permanent teeth which can be directly correlated to brain development. Brain development and tooth development appear to be parallel. This research was reported in 1994 at the International Society for fluoride research at a conference in Beijing which linked dental fluorosis to lower IQ. Conversely, iodine and PQQ raise IQ levels.*

And finally, a former toxicologist at the Harvard Forsyth Dental research Institute found that fluoride was more potent than lead in negatively impacting the behavior of animals. This study was published in the *Journal of Neurotoxicology*.†

It's quite clear that chronic ingestion of fluoride from drinking water has not been proven safe or effective, and there is ample evidence of harm from drinking fluoridated water.

So, what can you do to rectify the effects of fluoride in your environment? **Here are some very specific things you can do to help yourself:**

- **Stop using fluoridated anything,** including fluoride treatments from your dentistry team.
- **Many medications also contain fluoride.** Check the ingredients list. Anything that starts with a fluoro- has fluoride in it.
- **Increase your levels of B vitamins,** especially riboflavin, B2 since these vitamins increase fluoride excretion.
- **Increase your supplementation of R-lipoic acid;** it is a mercury chelator.
- **Never, ever drink treated municipal tap water.** Chlorine destroys vital lactobacillus needed in your gut. It's also full of everything the masses have thrown down their toilets.

---

* Jorge Flechas, MD, IAOMT, Annual Spring Meeting lecture notes.

† Budapest Study.

- **Increase your daily iodine levels.** You need at least 12.5 milligrams a day. Take Iodoral.
- **Use Celtic sea salt**—and use it on everything. As I said earlier, organic sea salt is not the problem; processed table salt is. This "good" salt is essential for proper body mineralization, cellular function, alkalization, and increasing cellular membrane voltage.
- **Increase your oral pH** by using an alkalinizing water machine. This destroys the harmful bacteria in the biofilm on your teeth and decreases acidic attack on your enamel. You may also brush with baking soda.

The Politics of the Food Industry and the GMO Dilemma

My youngest daughter, Angela, continually reminds me that Monsanto's crusade to gain better crop yields may well be a gigantic ploy to control our food supply and the health of our nation. "Ridiculous," you say? Well, consider this: 100 percent of the world's wheat crop is now genetically modified, and Monsanto is in the GMO business. But what's so bad about GMO foods? Let's look at a few revealing facts. Toxicology expert Don Huber explains:

> It is well-documented that . . . having that foreign plant gene inserted reduces the capability of that plant to take up nutrients. Then, when you apply the chemical glyphosate, you have a further compounding effect in reducing the efficiency of the plants at rates as low as 12 grams per acre.

The efficiency Dr. Huber refers to is the efficiency of producing the natural nutrients in the crops. This means there is virtually no nutritional value in many GMO foods.*

Another side effect of GMO production of foods is the way in which plants resist things like insect infestation. By disrupting the pests' digestive systems, the insects are unable to eat the plants. So, it doesn't take much imagination to make a potential connection to the dramatic increase in digestive problems among Americans.

According to Scott Laird at the Center for Disease Control, more than 57 million people in the United States visit hospitals and doctors every year due to digestive issues. Something like 70 to 80 percent of your immune system is located in your gut-associated lymphoid tissue (GALT) which is why the proper functioning of your GI tract is so critical. And anything that interferes with this system is a problem.

Refined Sugar, The Modern-Day Toxin

When it comes to proper functioning of the body, one other nearly ubiquitous substance interferes with good health in just about every way possible. Refined

---

* PPNF, *Journal of Health and Healing*: Fall 2017, https://price-pottenger.org/.

processed sugar is likely the most all-encompassing, nearly unavoidable toxin in our food environment today. It is what I call the modern-day toxin.

Sugar being eight times more addictive than cocaine complicates the job of reducing intake. Avoiding sugar is not just a matter of willpower. It is a matter of breaking a cycle of addiction, just as surely as freeing oneself from drugs or alcohol. But fleeing sugar addiction is crucial for good health.

Sugar shuts down the immune system and feeds cancer through a process called glycolysis. It also keeps insulin levels high which, as I've said already, causes you to become fat and stay fat. As a result, it is best to avoid refined sugars, and substitute other sources such as, monk fruit, coconut sugar, honey, jaggery, xylitol and D-ribose. Although it may be daunting to stay away from all sugar, you might as well know the truth about what you're fighting. So, as overwhelming as it may be, I've included below an unabridged list of what to avoid. The more you can keep away from these types of sugars, the better off you'll be.

This includes artificial sweeteners (yes, these often have chemicals as bad or worse than sugar itself—including those that claim to be "okay" like Splenda and Equal). These are things to watch out for:

- Anything that has high fructose corn syrup (HFCS) in it
- Cake, cookies, pies (they also contain trans-plastic fats)
- Candy
- Milk chocolate (cacao/dark chocolate is all right, but it must be at least 72 percent cacao)
- Almost all yogurt, including frozen yogurt
- Ice cream (unless it is made from raw milk)
- Jams and jellies
- Ketchup
- Molasses (blackstrap molasses is okay in small amounts)
- Soda (diet drinks are even worse than those with sugar)
- Sucrose

In general, anything that says "modified" on the label, put it back on the shelf. The battle against sugar also involves some intrigue. The "enemy" infiltrates our food in substances that are not specifically called "sugar." Here's a list of sugar additives to watch out for:

- Modified corn syrup
- Modified cornstarch
- Corn syrup
- Corn sugar (a euphemism for HFCS)
- Tapioca syrup
- Maltodextrin

- Dextrin
- Dextrose
- Acesulfame-k
- Fructose
- Glucose
- Invert glucose
- Invert sugar
- Lactose
- Maltose
- High maltose corn syrup
- Sorbitol
- Sorghum
- Fruit juice concentrate

So, once you've done all the avoiding you can, what positive action can you take? I'm glad you asked. You need to understand and pay attention to glycemic index and glycemic load (see chapter 7).

The Safe Sugars List

The list of safe sugars is shorter than the list of unsafe sugars, so it takes a little work to make sure you're eating the healthy alternatives. That being the case, I recommend that you take the safe sugars list with you when you go shopping.

These sugars are not made from corn, nor are they modified chemically or genetically. As a result, they are much healthier because your cells recognize their chemical composition and can use them as building blocks for various parts of the cell organelles. They can also fit into cellular-wall membrane receptors, like a lock and key mechanism. So, here they are:

- Sugar in the Raw (natural cane sugar) and coconut sugar
- Xylitol (use sparingly)
- D-ribose (great for your heart in that it is the template for the ATP molecule)
- D-mannose (great for your urinary health)
- Pure local honey (great for skin lesions)
- Stevia (popular, but use it sparingly—the others are better for you)
- Blackstrap molasses (packed with good minerals)
- Pure maple syrup (very alkaline—a good thing)
- Lo han guo, monk fruit
- Sulfoquinovose (SQ) This beneficial sugar feeds the good gut bacteria, acting like a prebiotic. (It's found mainly in vegetables.)*

---

* Hanson, B.T., Dimitri Kits, K., Löffler, J. et al. Sulfoquinovose is a select nutrient of prominent bacteria and a source of hydrogen sulfide in the human gut. ISME J 15, 2779–2791 (2021). https://doi.org/10.1038/s41396–021-00968–0.

Proper nutrient sugars are an integral part of the makeup of every one of your cell membranes. One of these sugars—xylitol—has some folks worried but please let me explain.

Xylitol is a five-carbon sugar alcohol that occurs naturally in fruits, vegetables, and woody plants, like birch. One of its key benefits is that it decreases the bacterial load especially with *Streptococcus mutans*, and *H.pylori*, the microorganism implicated in periodontal disease, bad breath, gastric and duodenal ulcers, and even stomach cancer.

Regular xylitol consumption improves periodontal disease by decreasing inflammation. The use of xylitol has shown to be associated with a reduction in nasal, sinus, and oropharyngeal infections. Studies in the *Journal of American Dental Association* have shown the use of xylitol-sweetened gum reducing cavities in children in a dose-dependent manner (i.e., the more gum chewed the fewer the cavities). One piece of xylitol chewing gum contains 3.5 grams of xylitol, and long-term studies have shown it to prevent dental caries. But: Do not give xylitol to your pets. They cannot digest this type of sugar, and it could be fatal.

Another non-sugar supplement that is beneficial in combating bone and teeth demineralization issues is Pearl Silica Drops® a trademarked, highly absorbable form of silica, which is in our new product line.

Xylitol is also safe for diabetics and helps with weight loss. So are D-Ribose and D-Mannose, which are 5-carbon sugars. They do not cause a significant rise in blood glucose and insulin levels, and this is important for those on an antiaging regimen. Having excess insulin can add fifteen years to your biological age, and the more table sugar you consume, the higher your insulin levels become.[*]

Research has shown that excess sugar and insulin are a lethal combination that causes diabetes and weight gain. **Here's a list of some of the clinically proven benefits of xylitol for use in dentistry:**

- Inhibits plaque and dental cavities
- Retards demineralization of tooth enamel
- Promotes remineralization of tooth enamel
- Increases salivary production
- Relieves "dry mouth"
- Protects salivary proteins (it is a protein stabilizer)
- Improves breath odor
- Reduces infections in the mouth and nasopharynx
- Reduces middle ear infections in pediatric patients

---

* Frank Shallenberger, MD, HMD, *Type 2 Diabetes Breakthrough; A Revolutionary Approach to Treating Type 2 Diabetes* (Basic Health Publications, Inc., 2005).

What's more, xylitol helps improve osteoporosis and increases bone mineral density (BMD). In several double-blind studies, xylitol is showing promising results in raising BMD. This is extremely significant because, according to figures compiled by the Academy of Orthopedic Surgeons, osteoporosis causes some 1.5 million fractures in the United States each year at a cost approaching $10 billion. In this regard, xylitol is especially good news for women since they tend to develop osteoporosis four times more often than men.*

Scientists propose that xylitol's bone density enhancing properties are due to its ability to promote intestinal absorption of calcium. Calcium absorption is impaired with aging, so even though the cost of xylitol may seem to be more than commercial sugars, it clearly represents a savings due to its many health benefits. There does not appear to be a toxic dose of xylitol, either. Remember: never let pets eat xylitol. People have safely taken up to 400 grams daily without significant ill effects. (High doses, however, have been shown to cause diarrhea, at least initially.)

The Benefits of Clean Water

Our body is made up of about 75 percent water, your brain bioplasm is about 85 percent water, and your blood is about 85 percent water. So, consuming clean water is the first best thing you can do. Water from an uncontaminated stream or deep well is full of minerals and, therefore, alkaline. This is desirable because it means the water contains electrons your body can use in the metabolic process. On the other hand, putting chlorine or fluoride into water causes it to become acidic and toxic, and anything acidic is an electron stealer (alkaline = electron donor).†

Water is a carrier of minerals, a solvent, a nutrient transport system, an electrical messaging system, a lubricant, a coolant, a heat bank, and a voltage storage facility. You get the picture, right? Also, consuming clean water has the following further benefits:‡

- Suppressing your appetite
- Reducing fat deposits in your body
- Relieving fluid retention problems
- Assisting in the metabolizing of stored fat
- Reducing sodium buildup in your body
- Helping to maintain proper muscle tone

* Rallie McCallister, MD, *The Benefits of Xylitol* (white paper).

† Dr. Masaru Emoto, http://www.flaska.eu/water-structuring/pioneers-of-water-research/dr-masaru-emoto; Dr. Nina Aksyonova-Walsh, http://www.keycompounding.com/spring-liver-detox/.

‡ Dr. Thomas Lokensgard, The Importance of Water, protocol, http://www.drlokensgard.com/shop.

- Diluting toxins in your cells
- Ridding your body of waste and toxins
- Relieving constipation

How do you get clean water that provides these benefits? If possible, get it right out of the ground. Water from the ground contains electrons. Most tap water has toxic levels of copper, hormones, every drug imaginable, and other stuff you don't really want to know about, and not all of that is filtered out. Even the good water needs to be stored in glass, not plastic, bottles. Use ozonated water or purchase a Kangen-water alkaline machine or a Berkey filtration system.*

You must drink water that restores and maintains a healthy mineral balance because this increases the voltage in your cells' bipolar lipid membrane. If you drink distilled water, you absolutely must add minerals.

To check your water's health level, you can test it with a voltmeter. If the voltmeter shows a minus voltage or a pH above 7.1, the water is an electron donor. If the voltmeter shows a plus voltage, or a pH below 6.9, the water is an electron stealer. You want water that is a donor of electrons.†

In chapter 1, I told you about my journey and that my study of whole-body medicine began in the mouth. After all, my field of endeavor is dentistry, first and foremost, so I'd like to explain more now about what makes the mouth such an important indicator of health and wellness. Let's start with sleep apnea and its relation to oxygen consumption.

* Laird Wellness; et al., https://rumble.com/v4cd2i0-how-to-make-immune-boosting-water.html.

† Tennant, *Healing Is Voltage.*

CHAPTER 10

OSA and Insomnia—Why Can't I Sleep?

Few things are as important as a good night's sleep. Waking up in the morning feeling fully refreshed and alert for the day is essential. Yet far, far too many people seldom experience this simple pleasure that is also essential to good health.

An adult needs an average of seven to eight hours of quality sleep per night in order for the body to adequately restore itself. Yet studies suggest that only about 35 percent of Americans consistently get this amount of rest. That means two thirds of us are chronically getting too little rest at night. In most cases, this is simply because we are under too much stress, our sympathetic nervous system is dominant, and our hormones, especially our neurotransmitters, are all out of whack. Work and other family activities squeeze what time is left out of the rest of our busy schedules.

OBSTRUCTIVE SLEEP APNEA (OSA)

For many others, though, lack of restful sleep is due to some form of obstructive sleep apnea (OSA),The causative agents are generally hormonal and neurotransmitter imbalances, especially increased cortisol, due to our dear old friends, stress and aging. OSA is a life-threatening condition as it is the cessation of breathing while one is asleep.

In 2004, OSA was at least partially to blame for the death of one of sports' leading figures, Reggie White, an NFL Hall of Fame Defensive Lineman, at forty-three years of age. OSA, in Reggie White's case, contributed to his death, which was a huge loss for all of us. He was a stellar player and the pillar of a Christian man.

If you are not sleeping well nor reaching REM sleep, then you are not secreting adequate amounts of human growth hormone (HGH), processing your short-term memory into long-term memory, nor detoxifying your liver, all of which take place during REM or deep sleep. Chances are great that oxygen deprivation would certainly be problematic. You need to have a sleep apnea test performed called a polysomnogram test.

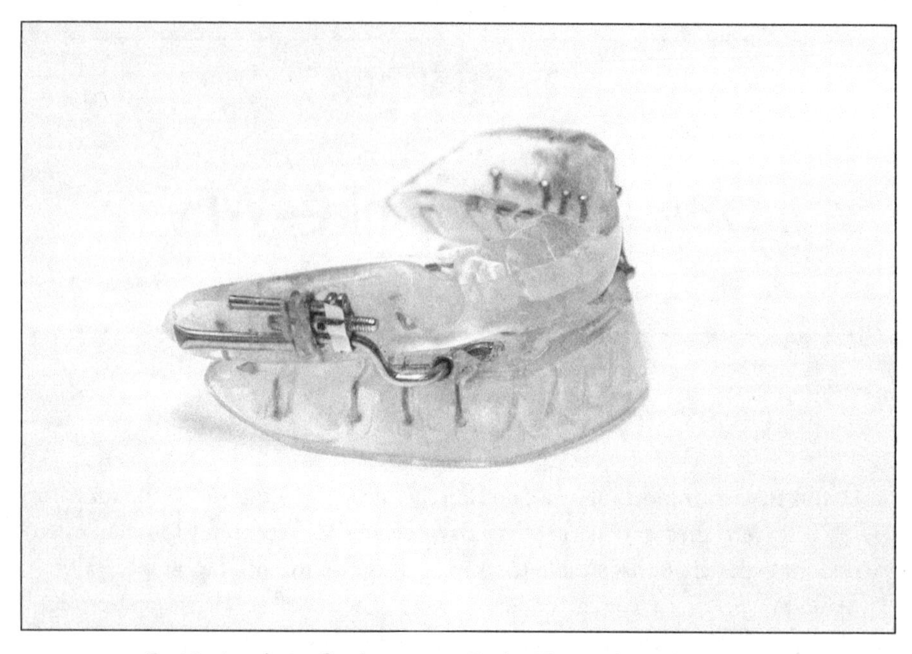

Positioning device for sleep apnea. Credit: Vinicius Vieira De Souza.

This sleep test will help determine your hypopnea index which will let you know whether you have mild, moderate, or severe OSA. If it's determined that you have mild to moderate sleep apnea, an OSA dental appliance that positions your jaw forward can be custom made for you instead of an obtrusive and noisy CPAP machine. If you have severe apnea, a combination of a CPAP machine and a dental appliance may be used.

Untreated OSA can be deadly, as in Reggie White's case, so know the dangers and seek treatment right away.

Please note: If you have had or are contemplating having a genetic SNPS test done, check your GAD levels. If you have a GAD polymorphism in your DNA profile, you may be unable to convert glutamic acid into GABA, which will inhibit the ability to stay asleep.

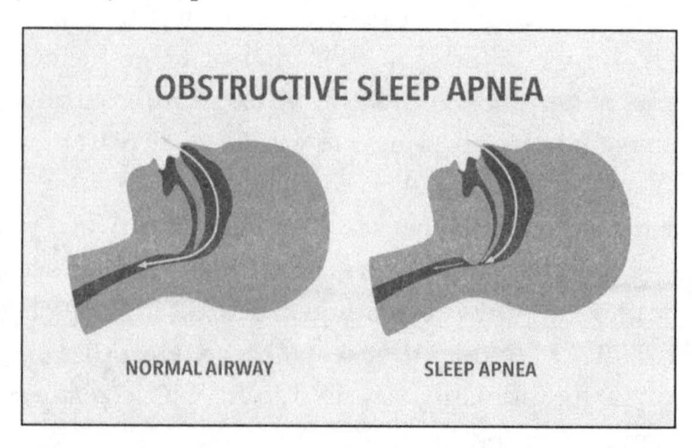

Depiction of obstructive sleep apnea. Credit: Blueastro.

Arrested Rest

Insomnia is the inability to sleep when sleep should normally occur, and this normal pattern of rest can be truncated in a variety of ways. People who struggle with insomnia generally experience one or more of these sleep disturbances:

- Difficulty falling asleep at night
- Waking too early in the morning
- Waking frequently throughout the night

Insomnia may stem from a disruption of the body's circadian rhythm, an internal clock that governs the timing of hormone production, sleep, body temperature, BPH, and other functions. While occasional restless nights are normal, prolonged insomnia can interfere with daytime function, concentration, and memory.

Insomnia is also associated with other health and lifestyle risks. People who have insomnia on a regular basis are at an increased risk of substance abuse, motor vehicle accidents, headaches, and depression. Research indicates that 50 percent of the US adult population suffers from sleep difficulties and as many as 35 percent struggle with such difficulties for at least one year. And of the one out of three people who have insomnia, only 20 percent ever bring it to the attention of their physicians.

If you manifest one of the insomnia patterns noted above, you can confirm whether your situation constitutes insomnia if you also have one or more of the following resultant symptoms:

- Not feeling refreshed after sleep
- Inability to sleep despite being tired
- Daytime drowsiness, fatigue, or irritability
- Difficulty concentrating and impaired ability to perform normal activities
- Anxiety as bedtime approaches

Fortunately, there are some healthy and effective ways to overcome insomnia.

Treat Yourself to a Good Night's Sleep

Although the standard knee-jerk-reaction treatment for insomnia is for a physician to prescribe one of the aggressively marketed "solutions" such as Ambien or other popular sleeping pills, by now I hope you know that these nonsolution solutions are yet another example of Band-Aid medicine. The good news, of course, is that there are truly healthful treatments that address the whole-body conditions required in order to sleep well. In fact, there are so many excellent options for treatment that it's astounding that doctors don't avail themselves of these methods. You can see from the list below that, with a little effort, you can find a solution that is right for you. Because so many options exist (and you hopefully won't have to do all of them), it is especially beneficial to work with a health practitioner to explore what you need.

There are many insomnia treatment aids to help you sleep. The list below is not exhaustive.*

1. 5-HTP
2. SaBio, a GABA agonist
3. Skullcap
4. PEMF mat for 30 minutes per day (I use an i-MRS mat)
5. Valerian root
6. Coenzyme Q10 (100 mg)
7. Phosphatidyl choline (3000 mg)
8. Remtyme
9. L-theanine (from green tea leaves; 50 mg generates calming effect on alpha brain waves)
10. Magnesium† (three to seven 50 mg capsules at night)
11. Chamomile extract (100 mg)
12. Lemon balm (50 mg)
13. Passion flower (4 percent vitexin, 25 mg)
14. Hops (25 mg)
15. Warm glass of raw whole milk or plant-based milk
16. DHA-EPA (1 to 3 grams)
17. Melatonin (60 mg) Start low and increase slowly, it is big-time cancer treatment
18. Serotonin
19. Cranio-electrical stimulation (30 minutes)
20. Inositol (500 mg one hour before bedtime)
21. *Griffonica simplicifola* (raises 5-HTP levels, increases synthesis of serotonin, and often reduces migraine headaches)
22. Alteril, a sleep aid containing L-tryptophan
23. L-arginine (3 to 7 grams). Or you can use L-citrulline, if you are over forty years of age
24. Oral-micronized progesterone or pregnenelone
25. Phosphatidyl Serine (decreases cortisol levels)

In addition to what you do, what you don't do is just as important. Avoiding all sugar and foods containing sugar is crucial. This includes aspartame, sucralose

---

* Dr. Thomas Lokensgard, So, Why Can't I Sleep, protocol, http://www.drlokensgard.com/shop.

† https://lairdwellness.com/collections/optiyourx-supplements.

(Splenda), and other sugar substitutes. These are neuro-excitotoxins, and they increase glutamate levels in the brain. Sucralose and Splenda, specifically, are suspects in the causation of hypothyroidism.

As part of addressing insomnia, you should also find out whether or not you have OSA. If you do, you must correct that problem because sleep apnea can interrupt your healthy sleep up to three hundred times in a single night. It destroys the effectiveness of your sleep, even if you sleep for eight full hours. For moderate apnea treatment, I strongly recommend an MRA-positioner dental appliance. In addition, lowering stress levels will help you sleep. This means not only lifestyle stress but also environmental stress.

You need to sleep with no lights and no electromagnetic radiation (i.e., cell phone and Wi-Fi waves). You should also make it a point to relax and read something boring before going to bed.

Finally, you'll want to reduce your caffeine intake, stay away from statin drugs (such as Zocor and Lipitor), and avoid alcohol of all kinds. It may make you drowsy at times, but alcohol interferes with the body's natural sleep mechanism and bolsters the CNS.*

* Woeller, *Resolving Chronic Stress Disorders.*

PART THREE

Solutions to Common Health Problems

CHAPTER 11

The Fattening of America

In the 1960s, President Johnson declared the "War on Poverty," and a couple of decades later, the medical industry started an undeclared "War on Dietary Fat." The simplistic thinking of the time was that eating fat made us fat. Both "wars" have been monumental failures and have contributed to the decline in our social culture, family structure, and our health, as they have cost America trillions of dollars with nothing to show for their noble efforts except obesity, debt, societal breakdown, and an insurance-controlled "disease care system" with a massive out-of-control synthetic food and death industry that's destroying our health.

And they are still wrong, espousing the brilliant government food pyramid, which is completely upside-down, along with the promotion of the low-fat, high-sugar diet. Ask any health coach, antiaging doctor, or fitness trainer.

I recall a former television commercial claiming that Honey Nut Cheerios were actually good for my heart. Really? And yet another commercial told me that "good parents" fed their kids Pop-Tarts for breakfast. Both claims were news to me. I was shocked (but not terribly surprised).

Have you ever read the labels to see what's in "junk" like Cheerios and Pop-Tarts? You probably wouldn't recognize most of the ingredients, but my rule of thumb is that if you can't pronounce the ingredient list, your liver and immune system probably don't know what to do with the ingredients either. Which means that if your body cannot process or metabolize the ingredients, it has to either store them or break them down, and then eliminate them. Eliminating them is a lot of work for the body, and storing leads to the problems we're talking about in this chapter.

The Lowdown on Low-Fat

Just as the commercial food industry and agribusiness giants, along with the FDA, USDA and American Heart Association, brought us the low-fat diet myth, they are fully vested in providing products that can be preserved for decades—on the shelf or in the fridge—with literally no nutritive food value at all. They've given us what I call over-consumptive undernutrition. Their boxed, canned, frozen, bagged, irradiated, hyper-processed, over-preserved, microwaveable, bioengineered food sources also have a common thread running through them all: fake sugar. And lots of it.

Our foods are processed and refined, synthetized and modified, calorie-packed or calorie-free (both bad), high- and low-glycemic concoctions masquerading under an assortment of trade and chemical names. And likely the most common and arguably worst culprit of all are the favorite consumables of way too many people: Soft drinks. Why? One reason: high fructose corn syrup (HFCS). Think cellular poison.

The commercial soft drink manufacturers have invested billions in advertising and have created some of the most successful marketing campaigns in American history. For many people, soft drinks are the single biggest source of sugar in their diet. Each brand can contain up to 10 to 12 teaspoons of sugar per serving. It would be bad enough if it were simply real sugar, but it's worse—much worse. The sugar in soft drinks is a liquid form of sugar called HFCS—high fructose corn syrup.*

The only drink alternative that's worse for you is the one they've spent billions more trying to make you think is better for you. I'm referring, of course, to diet soft drinks. They've even convinced countless people that drinking diet pop will help you lose weight. Nothing could be further from the truth. To make my point, let me enumerate some of the effects soft drinks have on your body.

1. **Soft drinks are hard on your health, skeleton, teeth, and weight.** Soft drinks contain caffeine, carbonation, refined sugars—or worse, sugar substitutes—food additives, such as artificial coloring, flavoring, and preservatives with little to no vitamins or other essential nutrients. They cause your blood sugar to skyrocket, and this causes insulin signaling that drives sugar into the cells to store the sugar as fat. This contributes to nonalcoholic fatty liver disease.†
2. **Consumption of soft drinks in high quantities—especially by children—is responsible for many health problems.** The documented list includes tooth decay, nutritional depletion, obesity, type 2 diabetes, heart disease, and depletion of calcium which can result in early osteoporosis, cognitive dysfunction, and even some forms of cancer.
3. **Soft drinks "poison" us with sugar.** Most soft drinks contain high amounts of refined sweeteners, yet the USDA recommends sugar consumption in a two-thousand-calorie diet be limited to a daily allotment of ten teaspoons of added sugar (which is still way too high in

* Janice Lorigan, *High Fructose Corn Syrup and the Fibromyalgia Connection* (AuthorHouse, 2007).

† Roger Deutsch and Rudy Rivera, MD, *Your Hidden Food Allergies are Making You Fat* (Prima Lifestyles, 2002) 152–55.

this author's opinion). As I mentioned above, many soft drinks contain more than that amount in just one can!

4. **The refined sweeteners and simple sugars in soft drinks force the pancreas into overdrive.** Your pancreatic beta cells are called upon to produce and release insulin, a hormone that empties the sugar from your bloodstream into all the tissues and cells for usage. This raises the blood insulin levels beyond the norm and can lead to depression of the immune system and a weakening of your ability to fight disease, and it also leads to extra weight gain. Because insulin is a fat storage hormone, when your blood sugar levels remain elevated (such as what happens when you regularly drink soda pop), you get fat, and you stay fat. All because insulin is merely doing what it is meant to do: Storing sugar in your fat cells for future energy. But when there is no energy expenditure (as in "couch potatoism"), your body turns the cellular sugar to fat, especially into triglycerides. This is one of the reasons why excess sugar consumption can result in elevated risks for heart disease and cancer.
5. **Diet sodas contain artificial sweeteners such as aspartame, sucralose, or saccharin which pose a big threat to your health.** Saccharin, for instance, has been found in some studies, to be carcinogenic (cancer-causing).
6. **Diet drinks increase glutamate production in the brain.** Too much glutamate actually destroys brain cells.
7. **Nutrasweet (known as aspartame and present in most diet drinks) is a well-known chemical neuro-excitotoxin.** It's a chemical that fools the brain into thinking blood sugar is elevated, causing even more insulin to be secreted, leading to more carbohydrate loading. Aspartame studies have found it is closely linked to obesity. We are destroying our kids with this stuff.
8. **Splenda (known as sucralose, also present in many diet drinks) is a noncaloric artificial sweetener made from sucrose.** Although it is six hundred times sweeter than sugar, the body cannot absorb it. As a result, it increases body weight and disrupts and reduces beneficial intestinal bacteria.
9. **Beverages with bubbles contain phosphoric acid.** Phosphate can severely deplete blood calcium levels, a key component of the bone matrix. This increases the risk of osteoporosis and dental decay. It also reverses the flow of nutrients in the DFTS.

Quite a mess we're in, isn't it? But who's to blame?

The Battle with Food Manufacturers

Remember the paradigm-shifting seminar I mentioned earlier? I've thought about this for many years now and have concluded this gentleman was well ahead of his time. The food processing industry creates the synthetic, artificial, sugar-laden, genetically modified, obesogenic, cancer-causing foods that have set the stage for chronic degenerative disease, including dental decay. And the food industry is still lining our grocery shelves with this garbage.

That's why you must know which 20 percent of the food supply in the grocery store is actually fit for your consumption. Certainly, the manufacturers aren't going to tell you. In order to take full responsibility for our own good health, it's up to you and me to become well-informed, educated consumers because what we eat matters—big-time and for the long term.

I talked earlier about insulin signaling and how it contributes to obesity, but there's another crucial side to the fat equation as well. It centers around the fat-burning hormone known as glucagon. When blood sugar levels are low (i.e., when you are truly hungry), this hormone signals stored sugar (glycogen) to come out of the cell and be burned as fuel, but here's the problem: When blood sugar levels remain high (like when we eat typical American levels of sugar), glucagon never gets a chance to come to the rescue, and your body never gets a chance to burn the fat.

This is why sipping on soda pop and sugary treats all day long is a really, really, really bad idea. Sugar levels stay up all day long, and no fat gets burned.

Another part of the food-education process is to realize that sugar is also hidden in many—often surprising—places, such as low-fat foods. When you see "low-fat" on any grocery store item, move on. It's almost always code for "high sugar."

Years ago, science informed us that consuming fat would make you fat. In a simplistic way, that would seem to make sense. Eat fat, get fat—right? Wrong. Eating fats does not make you fat. Again, like with refined salt, it must be the right kind. But eating sugar certainly does make you fat and helps keep you fat. As for the good fats, omega-3s are essential for proper brain and cardiovascular functioning and for healthy weight management.

It's the sugar component in foods that causes an increase in triglycerides, metabolic syndrome, and glycation (also known as advanced glycation end products, or AGEs).*

Glycation is the process which causes stiffening of the arterioles and neurofibrillary tangles in the brain (Alzheimer's disease), and it is also bad for your skin. Sugar is highly inflammatory and very acidic (remember how bad those two things are?).

* Life Extension, *The Science of a Healthier Life, Glucose: The Silent Killer,* Journal Article (January 2011).

Sugar is also hidden in all manufactured food products (see my list of Hidden Sugars, Life Rejuvenation Program in Appendix 10). Simply stated: If you consume lots of sugar and empty calories in soft drinks or energy drinks, you will gain weight and become insulin resistant. It's called the metabolic syndrome.

The healthy food consumption piece of the modern American medical paradigm is essentially missing in action. Your body is an amazing, intricate machine that runs on proper fuel, just like a high-end sports car. Your immune system does not recognize artificial colorings, flavorings, synthetic pharmaceuticals, trans fats, fillers, and many of the other mythical biologically antithetical substances we cram into our bodies.

Each cell in the human body has a remarkable God-ordained, preprogrammed genetic ability to heal itself, if given the right environment and the correct nutrients. That's what naturopathy is all about. However, the generally accepted "symptom management practice" of contemporary medicine ignores this basic fact and has led us down an expensive and dangerous road to chronic illness and disease.

This is a big factor, for instance, in the widespread propensity these days toward allergy problems. And guess what common sugar substance (so common that it is found in most sweetened foods) is the biggest offender? The nearly ubiquitous HFCS—high fructose corn syrup.

But there's some really good news for people (like you) who learn to eat in "traditional" ways. It's been shown that those who eat traditional diets (i.e., non-processed, unadulterated foods) experience a drastically reduced incidence of cancer, obesity, fibromyalgia, osteoporosis, tooth decay, adult-onset diabetes (now occurring in nine-year-old kids), and increasing cardiovascular disease, just to name a few.*

The fact is: If we stop eating processed, fast foods, soda pop, and sugar-laden (especially HFCS) sweets and choose fresh, organic fruits, vegetables, nuts, grass-fed meats, wild-caught fish, and GMO-free plants, we will benefit from dramatic health and weight improvements in an astoundingly short time. It only takes one generation to screw things up. Weston A. Price and Frank Pottenger figured this out in the 1920s.

The Low-Fat Diet Myth

The problem with the low-fat-diet craze is that we took out the healthy omega-3 fats and added refined sugar along with omega-6 trans-plastic fat—lots of it—into the mix. This has become an unmitigated disaster, as trans-fatty fats cause plastic cellular membranes which don't allow proper cellular membrane transport. Even

* Weston A. Price, DDS, *Nutrition and Physical Degeneration, 1939* (Price-Pottenger Nutrition Foundation Publishing, 2008).

as I write this, I still see plenty of commercials espousing the merits of the low-fat diet.

So, what, exactly, is wrong with the low-fat (high-sugar) diet? To begin with, it is based on an altogether erroneous foundation, the false belief that eating fat makes you fat. We've already stated that fat consumption doesn't cause obesity; sugar consumption does.

The low-fat diet, however well-intentioned, is loaded with highly refined, non-nutritional sugars that raise postprandial (after meal) sugar levels. As described earlier, it is the insulin-signaling triggered by elevated sugar levels that causes you to pack on the pounds.

Insulin is a fat-storage hormone that signals your cells to store excess sugar as triglycerides, which contributes to cardiovascular disease, aging, and obesity. High insulin levels also cause brain inflammation and a laundry list of other issues. After-meal sugar spikes, for instance, cause the retinal, kidney, and cardiovascular, endothelial damage that contributes to our inflammatory health problems by keeping you chronically inflamed.

Food manufacturers sold us a bag of "toxic goods" as we were told time and again that it's the calories that matter. Then, by dumping a bunch of zero-calorie, highly neurotoxic fake sugar (which can be produced very profitably), they led us to believe we would lose weight. But what has really happened as a result? In the last half century in America, we have seen the greatest increase in weight gain in the history of the planet. No footnote needed here, just look around you.

Calories simply have a lesser impact on weight, especially compared to the effect of insulin signaling. Low-fat diets are full of sugar, and plastic obesogenic, endocrine disruptors—i.e., the stuff on the labels whose names you can't pronounce. When you eat it, your body is left to deal with all the toxins in these packaged concoctions and has to work overtime to rid your cells of the toxicity, overloading your liver.

Adipocyte cells have five basic ways to handle the toxin overload:

1. **Dilution of the intracellular fluid** to neutralize the toxins in your cells. Your cells swell up with water in order to dilute the toxins.
2. **The solution to pollution is dilution**, and your body operates on this principle.
3. **Increasing the size and number of fat cells**, known as adipocytes. This process is called adipogenesis, the growth of new fat cells.
4. **Raising your insulin levels** to combat the continual sugar surges. This leads to insulin resistance, diabetes and fatty liver disease (your liver stores the sugar as fat).
5. **Producing antibodies (allergies)** to combat the unrecognized toxins, causing autoimmune dysfunction.

To make matters worse, the fats that have been removed in low-fat diets typically are the healthy omega-3 fats that happen to be protective of the cardiovascular and nervous system, and they have been replaced by highly inflammatory omega-6 vegetable oils! Grocery stores have aisles of this inflammatory and unhealthy vegetable oil. Healthy fats are essential for neurological and cardiovascular health, as well as efficient energy expenditure.

The key is the correct fatty acid ratio, not the elimination of fats altogether. This is measured by the bio-inflammatory AA/EPA omega-3 fatty acid index. Omega-3, -7, and -9 fatty acids are vitally important to prevent fanning the flames of chronic inflammation.* The now-standard way of thinking about what makes us fat is one of the things you need to be concerned with by taking a wiser approach. Otherwise, you'll keep doing the same, anti-healthful dietary practices that are fattening us to death. Do that, and you're on your way to winning the interior battle for your health.

The goal of the mega-giant food industry is twofold:

1. To make food that tastes good and is addictive ("High sugar content"—we now know that sugar is more addictive than cocaine; some experts say by eight times).
2. To make inexpensive foodstuffs that last on the shelf for years.

By contrast, we're designed to eat real food that will spoil because of its enzyme content. If the bugs aren't interested in eating it, you shouldn't be, either. The key is to eat whole food, but eat it before it spoils. I believe we are designed to eat lots of varieties of food, say 120 different food types per season, to eat less (CR) than we typically do, and to eat more slowly than we usually do. I think that too many of us eat the same old, same old, seven to ten foodstuffs each and every day with little to no variation.

---

* Stephen T. Sinatra, MD, FACC, FACN, CNS, CBT, *Heart, Health, and Nutrition* Newsletter, https://heartmdinstitute.com/.

CHAPTER 12

Controlling Chronic Constipation

In the United States, chronic constipation is *the* most common gastrointestinal complaint. Yet the generally prescribed remedy—increased ingestion of fiber—has been shown to be ineffective in 80 percent of all patients treated for increased bowel transit time (medicalese for constipation). With a lack-of-success rate like this, something is wrong. People who are willing to look beyond the simplistic, bulk-up-on-fiber protocol, though, will find some very promising options for resolving this issue. Making sure your colon is healthy is important, much like keeping your mouth healthy, because gut health is another crucial component of whole-body health. Remember that if you are not eliminating on a daily basis, you are becoming more toxic by the day.*

Attack the Cause, Solve the Problem

The successful conclusion of your digestive process—i.e., excretion of bowel waste—depends on the proper working of the peristaltic action of your colonic system. Peristalsis refers to the series of rhythmic, involuntary muscular contractions that move food through the intestines and lower colon. When the system is healthy, the final stage concludes with the ready ejection of waste material.

One of the primary causes of constipation is ineffective peristalsis, which results in impacted fecal material. When your bowels are not moving due to an incomplete or insufficient contractile pattern of the muscles surrounding the intestines (especially the large colon), you have a problem. Getting rid of the fecal matter becomes difficult. And guess what? Lack of fiber is not necessarily the cause of this condition.

The good news is that the correct solution to this chronic situation is not much more complicated than "taking fiber," the simple "remedy" that oftentimes is not quite enough. By drinking the correct nutrients first thing upon waking in the morning, you can generate a wave of peristaltic action that will evacuate leftover fecal matter—usually within one to three hours.

---

* Life Extension, *The Science of a Healthier Life, Get Immediate Relief from Constipation*, Journal Articles (November/December 2013), 8.

Colon Nourishment

The even better news is that a variety of options exist for using the correct nutrients, and the reason this is important is that—unlike the one-treatment-fits-all fiber prescription—your protocol can be readily adjusted to fit the needs of your own body. Each of us operates slightly differently, so a little experimentation is necessary to determine the precise solution that will work for you. I'd suggest working with your practitioner.

Since a number of potential remedies are available, I've outlined a list of possibilities below. The first option to try is this:

- Use the recommended serving of LIFE EXTENSION Effervescent Vitamin C Magnesium Crystals
- In addition, take one or two tablespoons per day of buffered vitamin C powder

If that works for you, then you're good to go (so to speak). On the other hand, if you still have constipation problems after using the magnesium and vitamin C protocol, here are other suggestions to discuss with your healthcare provider:

- **ConcenTrace® by TraceMinerals®.** Take twenty-one drops per day to bowel tolerance. Reduce the number of drops if the dosage causes continued diarrhea. Add also six to ten drops of Pearl Silica Drops®.
- **Complete Cleansing Fiber Part 1 & 2 by TraceMinerals®.** This regimen is a "one stop shop" for bowel cleansing.
- **Bob's Red Mill Flaxseed.** Take two heaping tablespoons twice a day (morning and evening) with lots of water.
- **Sea salt.** Add ½ teaspoon to your water daily to maintain electrolytic balance (it's good for your heart also).
- ***Cascara sagrada.*** Take two or three capsules a day (with twelve ounces of water); as this is a powerful peristaltic rhythmic enhancer, you'll want to use it liberally every day.
- **Organic Bowel Cleanse.** A regimen of colon-cleansing herbs available from Renew Life.
- **3 Ballerina herbal tea.** While this encourages elimination, it should be used with caution. Stop taking it if diarrhea persists or you experience negative symptoms.
- **Magnesium sulfate or magnesium chloride.** Dosing at night will help you get to sleep faster while it works on your bowels. Also note that taking choline citrate will greatly increase the absorption of magnesium and could increase the advantage of this healing measure.

- **Magnesium citrate or malate** if taken in amounts of 1,000 milligrams or more. I would also suggest magnesium-L-threonate, 800 mg per day, as it crosses the BBB.
- **Drink the recommended daily amount of water** with all of these options (half your weight in ounces).

  As with most medical practices, I need to add a disclaimer on a few of the suggestions I've made. The nutrients listed below can cause diarrhea and so should be used with caution to minimize the presence of overly loose stools.
- **Powdered potassium** (vitamin K+). Since most of us are deficient in K+, though, the chance of K+ creating a problem is minimal.
- **Powdered vitamin B-5**
- **Powdered vitamin C** if using amounts in the range of 2,000 to 5,000 milligrams per day.
- **Pacific Coast pine bark** which contains cascarosides that boost the relaxation–contraction cycle of the colon.
- **Oregano oil** (to rid yourself of parasites) should be used for no more than two or three months at a time.

If you're interested in learning more about how all of these recommendations work and why, I have written protocols that are available on my website.[*] The Candida Conundrum protocol will explain how to rid yourself of yeast.[†] And speaking of yeast, that's what we need to talk about next. You'll be amazed at the consequences these little buggers can cause.[‡]

---

* Dr. Thomas Lokensgard, Protocols, http://www.drlokensgard.com/shop.

† Lokensgard, http://www.drlokensgard.com/shop, et al.

‡ Dr. Josh Axe, *Eat Dirt!* (HarperCollins Publishers, 2016).

CHAPTER 13

The Candida Conundrum

Candida is a family of fungi or yeasts that are virtually everywhere in our environment, on our skin, and in our intestines. When candida is present in moderate levels and the biological terrain is adequate, it does not negatively affect the body. If allowed to grow uncontrolled, however, it can wreak havoc on the body's physiology, and this overgrowth is rampant these days. An estimated 70 percent or more of the US population have a condition known as "chronic yeast infection" or candidiasis (thrush), but the condition is largely overlooked and underdiagnosed.

Medical lab reports and standard bloodwork often reveal little or nothing about candida, so in treating candida-related symptoms, doctors frequently default to prescribing antibiotics. The serious problem with this, though, is that antibiotics drive up the amount of yeast in the gastrointestinal tract and in the sinuses. While all doctors should know this, few pay attention, to the detriment of their patients.

CRC: The Candida-Related Complex

Every year, tens of thousands of people have experienced many seemingly unrelated symptoms that can't be explained by symptom-based conventional medicine. But there is a possible explanation: *Candida albicans.*

Candida interferes with the immune system by disrupting the natural suppressor cells (NSCs), also known as T-regulatory cells. These cells are the "brakes" that keep your immune system from attacking itself. Normally, NSCs comprise about 15 percent of a healthy immune system, but when yeast flares up, the proportion can drop to 1 percent or less. Once the yeast is treated, NSCs can rise to a normal level, and the immune system functions properly again.

In healthy people, the immune system prevents candida from growing out of control, but a compromised immune function can allow candida to proliferate, resulting in a condition called candidiasis, also called SIBO. This is often the problem behind an assortment of undiagnosed symptoms. In fact, adults and children who "get sick all the time," are fatigued, have allergies, endure repeated ear infections, have skin problems, or struggle with depression most likely have candida overgrowth. A common cause is consumption of too much sugar—which is a problem for most Americans.

A weakened immune system caused by gut dysbiosis can be caused by various factors, including the following:

- Antibiotic therapy overuse
- Alcohol
- Birth control
- Cancer
- Chemotherapy
- Cortisone or prednisone use
- Diabetes and metabolic syndrome
- Excessive sugar in the diet
- Infection
- Medications
- Obesity
- Poor digestive function, namely gut dysbiosis
- Poor nutrition
- Chlorinated water
- Stress

When candida overgrows, it can infect every organ and tissue in the body and may cause virtually every known symptom, ranging from oral thrush and anal itching to poor memory, joint pain, and dry skin. Yeast produces toxins called acetaldehydes that are chemically related to formaldehyde. These block lymphatic and neurological function and can also decrease collagen and energy production.

Unfortunately, diagnostic tests that can definitively tell whether or not you have candida overgrowth are not widely used by symptom-based medicine, and the antifungal drugs that are used are notoriously inadequate for controlling candidiasis. Tests are available, but your practitioner needs to be aware of them and the importance of checking for candida. See the Candida Questionnaire in the protocol section on my website.*

The Great Mimicker

Dr. Orian Truss, author of *The Missing Diagnosis* and *The Missing Diagnosis II*, coined the term "the great mimicker" to refer to the symptomatic issues created by candida. He observed that symptoms often send doctors and their patients on a wild-goose chase as yeast levels rise and fall. The technical term for this situation is poly-systemic candidiasis, but by any name, it is a troublesome condition

* Lokensgard, http://www.drlokensgard.com/shop.

that can cause multiple chemical sensitivities, allergies, and swollen mucous membranes, all of which can look like symptoms of some other problem.

Yeast causes this systemic problem because it produces a toxic load of more than seventy identifiable toxins. In response, the body begins producing antibodies. This triggers a chronic fungus infection that burrows into the GI tract, causing leaky gut syndrome and gut inflammation.*

When this happens, the intestinal wall becomes more porous, and undigested protein is forced through the gut wall. The gut intestinal epithelium normally consists of a tight junctional wall, but when this wall is breached, the yeast then moves into the bloodstream and lymphatic system. The white blood cells signaled by this process must break down the undigested, toxic, food particles in the blood and this sets off a myriad of allergic symptoms, due to the increased antibody production and cytokine release.

Chronic yeast and fungus overgrowth must be treated. It absolutely, positively must be eradicated from your system, including your own mouth. Candidiasis can be kept under control only by maintaining a healthy gastrointestinal tract—that is to say, a thicker gut mucosal lining. This is why taking probiotics, prebiotics, digestive enzymes, betaine hydrochloride, zinc, iodine, and colostrum, increasing Secretory IgA, taking *Saccharomyces boulardii* (a beneficial essential yeast), and managing sugar intake, along with stomach acid content, is vitally important.

Yeast loves mucosal linings, sinuses, and mucous membranes, and as part of its "fakery," yeast also produces false estrogenic compounds that signal to the body that it has adequate levels of estradiol. This little deception upsets estrogenic balance, which upsets many other things. One result is menstrual irregularities which can contribute to fertility problems. Fortunately, as you kill off yeast overgrowth, your autoimmune imbalance issues can improve. But in order to treat it, you have to know the enemy. Candida overgrowth is often mistaken for other issues, but there are ways to know exactly what you're dealing with.

Symptoms of Candidiasis

The best way to determine if you have a candida problem is to evaluate whatever array of symptoms that may be present. Taken together, they often point to candidiasis. Below is a list of symptoms to look for.

The first thing to look for is a yellowish coating on your tongue. Next are:

- Adrenal fatigue
- Athlete's foot
- Anxiety
- Bloating and gas

---

* Dr. Josh Axe, *Eat Dirt!* (HarperCollins Publishers, 2016).

- Consistent brain fog (also a key sign of mercury in your system, which means you should get amalgam fillings removed correctly and completely)
- Chronic fatigue, usually a lack of O_2 metabolism or mitochondrial dysfunction
- Congestion or a runny nose that remains chronic
- Frequent burning in the urinary tract
- Headaches and acne
- Hair falling out, also a thyroid issue
- Heartburn and GERD (very symptomatic and usually completely misdiagnosed by pharmaceutical-oriented doctors)
- Heartburn in the aging process is usually the result of too little—not too much—stomach acid
- Inability to lose weight
- Interstitial cystitis
- Lots of colds and rashes
- Lowered libido
- Ongoing IBS and vaginal yeast infections
- Rectal itching
- Sick feeling all the time

If you have several of these, then chances are extremely high that you have candida overgrowth in the mouth and small bowel, called small intestinal bowel overgrowth (SIBO).

You can also do a simple home test to confirm whether you have candida overgrowth. When you wake up in the morning, spit into a glass of clean water. Wait thirty minutes and then examine what has happened to the saliva in the glass. If it is floating on the surface and has grown tentacles or fingerlike projections that hang down into the water, then you have a candida problem.

And the Solution Is?

The three-word summary of how to get rid of candidiasis is to starve it out. To do that, here's the safe, natural, and straightforward seven-step candida solution recommended in Dr. Laurence Smith's helpful book[*]:

(For overall guidance on what to eat to combat candida, see the Anti-Candida Diet below.)

1. Avoid high-yeast foods.[†]

---

* Laurence Smith, and C. Norman Shealy, MD, *Is Candida Sabotaging Your Health?* (CreateSpace Independent Publishing Platform, 2014).

† http://www.webmd.com/diet /foods-high-in-yeast.

2. Avoid sugar, artificial foods, and additives.
3. Eat a low-carbohydrate diet (absolutely no refined sugars).
4. Keep a proper acid-alkaline balance. Regulating the body's pH balance can help control candidiasis.
5. Use SBO probiotics from Ancient Nutrition.* Probiotics are friendly intestinal bacteria that can fight candida, contribute to a healthy pH, and assist immune function. (Use *S. boulardii*, a beneficial yeast, also.)
6. Use Bifidobacterium and lactobacillus, along with digestive enzymes, to clear the yeast. (Hydrozyme, from Biotics Research.†)
7. Eliminate all wheat products, processed milk and meats, and gluten products.

In addition to managing your diet, the battle against candidiasis can be helped by supplementing with herbs and other nutrients such as these:

- Argentyn 23 (Nanotech silver hydro-sol)
- Coconut oil
- Black walnut hull
- Caprylic acid (a MCFA in coconut oil, breast milk, and butter, better than Nystatin)
- Echinacea
- Elecampane root
- Garlic
- Oregano leaf extract
- Pau d'arco (a plant found in the rain forest. Can be used as a tea, capsules, or ointment) ‡
- Proprionic acid
- Red raspberry leaf
- Sorbic acid
- Tea tree oil
- Selenium
- Vitamin D3
- Zinc
- Iodine, 12.5 mg per day
- Una de gato (Cat's Claw)
- Barberry root
- Bearberry leaf

---

* Ancient Nutrition, https://ancientnutrition.com/pages/probiotics-digestionAncientNutrition .com.

† Biotics Research, http://www.bioticsresearch.com/.

‡ Pau d'arco is contraindicated for pregnant or nursing women. Please consult with an herbalist or other healthcare professional when embarking on any herbal regimen.

- Candi Bactin-AR
- Candisol (this one supplement contains most of the products in this list)
- Grape seed extract
- Red thyme oil
- Rhizome extract
- Slippery elm bark
- Undecyclenic acid
- Goldenseal root
- Acerin
- Babul bark
- Swedish birch bark
- L-glutamine (unless you have cancer)

Lifestyle choices also have a lot to do with success in overcoming candidiasis. These are some particularly important habits when battling candida:

- Getting enough sleep
- Maintaining a positive attitude
- Enjoying the detoxification benefits of a sauna and massages
- Limiting intake of coffee, alcohol, and chlorinated water and drinks (chlorine destroys lactobacillus)

As you progress in your candida fight, you'll need to clean out the dead yeast in your system. It takes up to two or three weeks for the yeast to die off and newly laid yeast eggs to hatch, so you'll have to persist in order to overcome this cycle.

Here is the regimen for eliminating dead yeast:[*]

1. Enzyme therapy (candisol)
2. Cellulase (take on an empty stomach)
3. Hemicellulase (take on an empty stomach)
4. Xylanase (take on an empty stomach)
5. Beta-glucanase (take on an empty stomach)
6. Protease (optional)—take only with food to aid in protein digestion

You'll need to repeat this several times since the whole die-off process can take months. Be aware that your symptoms may get worse for up to a month, as the yeast begins to die off in twenty-one days. Then, after another twenty-one days, it may happen again as the budding yeast expires. This is known as a Herxsheimer's reaction, and is caused by the yeast die-off.

---

* http://www.naturessunshine.com/.

During your battle with candida, your diet plays a significant role and involves an array of do's and don'ts.

Although it's difficult to assemble an exhaustive list of beneficial foods, I've outlined below a range of foods that are helpful in the fight against candida. Fermented beans are a good source of protein, but watch out for lectins.

The "Go for It" List:

- Avocado (these are very calorie dense but an excellent source of healthy fats)
- Coconut oil (contains MCTs or medium-chain fatty acids)
- Organic frozen berries (eat with raw milk to balance the carbs)
- Non-starchy vegetables (such as broccoli, asparagus, cauliflower, etc.)
- Good fats (omega-3, omega-9, omega-7, and GLA or borage oil)
- Olive oil (omega-9)
- Most fish, must have scales and no bottom dwellers
- Most grass-fed meats (especially wild-caught game)
- Organic poultry
- Raw milk and dairy
- Non-processed rice milk
- Romaine lettuce
- Minute amounts of xylitol, D-ribose, D-mannose (manage your intake, though, because these can cause diarrhea)

Grains and legumes that do not contain gluten, such as:

- Amaranth (presoaked)
- All beans (except soy)
- Buckwheat
- Lentils (brown, red, and green)
- Millet
- Quinoa
- Split peas
- Almonds
- Cashews (contain a lot of lectins, so use minimally)
- Flaxseed
- Hazelnuts
- Filberts
- Pecans
- Pistachios
- Poppy seeds
- Pumpkin seeds

- Sesame seeds
- Sunflower seeds
- Walnuts

Soak certain seeds and nuts in order to deactivate the phytic acid content which binds up the needed mineral content in the seeds. For example, soaking almonds overnight or soaking sunflower and pumpkin seeds for a few hours before consumption can help reduce phytic acid levels and improve nutrient absorption.

The speed of your recovery and ultimate success in eliminating Candida also depends on how well you manage the "Don't List." Here's the rundown on what you should avoid while on the Candida-elimination protocol:

- Breads, buns, and pastries
- Cheese and anything containing processed cheese
- Coffee (because just 1 cup of coffee decreases one third of all good probiotics; replace coffee with high-quality protein and protein shakes with raw milk)
- Vinegar
- Cooking vegetables increases their carbohydrate value, so eat raw as much as possible.
- Fermented foods
- Mushrooms
- Sweets and sweeteners
- Mayonnaise and mustard
- Alcohol in any form—beer, wine, or liquor
- Antibiotics
- Refined sugars or foods of any kind that contain them
- Oranges and bananas
- Highly acidic foods or drinks
- Peanuts and peanut butter (contain aflatoxins, which are molds)
- Dairy products, except grass-fed butter
- Birth control pills (because they alter your hormonal balance)
- Chlorinated water
- Mildew or mold in your living space (use an air purifier/ionizer such as a Medi Air Purifier, to decrease mold; MS and COPD can also improve when you purify the air in your home.)

All this may sound complicated, and in truth, it's not simple. That's why I recommend that you work with a qualified professional to determine the best candida battle plan for you.

NATURAL YEAST FIGHTERS

When you have yeast in your body you will retain water. Water then enters your cells to dilute the toxins and you gain weight. People that have a buildup of toxic metals, especially mercury, in the gut will find it nearly impossible to rid themselves of candida.

You must get rid of the toxic metals first, or you'll never totally get rid of the yeast. Yeast is an often overlooked medical condition that can raise chaos with all of your bodily systems. It can take many months to get rid of this condition, but you must achieve a candida-free GI tract.

Here are some natural ways to control yeast overgrowth:

- Garlic, especially aged garlic
- Argentyn-23®, a silver hydrosol formulation made by Natural Immunogenics
- Biotin
- OxyMist® (Pearl Oral Health)
- Caprylic Acid
- Goldenseal
- Oregano, check out Biotics Research
- Lactoferrin, a subfraction of whey protein. Take 1 to 3 capsules daily with or without meals. Studies have shown lactoferrin inhibits gram-positive and gram-negative bacteria along with some yeasts and parasites.
- Tea tree oil
- Bifidobacterium, for large colon
- *Lactobacillus acidophilus*, for small intestine
- *Lactobacillus bifidum*
- Use HCL, hydrochloric acid, also known as betaine hydrochloride, from Biotics Research
- Pancreatic enzymes, from Biotics Research, called beta plus
- FOS, fructooligosaccharides, these are prebiotics that fuel the probiotics

Repair after the Battle's Won

The main casualty in the candida war is your gastrointestinal system, especially the liver. The harm done over time by candida, however, is repairable, and you're ready to start the process of gut repair once the candida has been eradicated. At this point, the "leaky gut" is what you need to heal.*

Consume soluble fibers such as apple pectin, SCFAs, and FOS. At the same time, you'll need to stay away from wheat and other products containing gluten as well as processed dairy foods. For any foods you've eliminated while combating

* Axe, *Eat Dirt.*

candida, you'll need to reintroduce them one at a time and monitor your symptoms, if any. Many of your food allergies will likely disappear, but you may also want to take an ALCAT test (see your practitioner for this) to see what food sensitivities you may still have.

Long-term supplementation will also help repair your gut. The foremost need, of course, is to rebuild your gut lining.

Once you've eliminated candida overgrowth and healed your gut, you'll be amazed at the difference in the way you feel. Managing your diet as outlined above may seem daunting, but you'll feel so much better that it will be motivating to maintain a healthier regimen of eating.[*, †, ‡, §]

---

* Life Extension, *The Science of a Healthier Life*, Journal Articles. *Disease Prevention and Treatment: Scientific Protocols That Integrate Mainstream and Alternative Medicine* (Life Extension Media, 4th edition, 2003), 409.

† Deanna Minnich, MD, *Whole Detox* (HarperOne, 2016).

‡ Sherry Rogers, MD, *Detoxify or Die* (Prestige Publishers, 2002).

§ Smith and Shealy, *Is Candida Sabotaging Your Health?*

CHAPTER 14

Heavy Metal and Whole-Body Detoxification

In chapter 9, we talked about the problem of living in a toxic world. To an extent, toxins are unavoidable, and as a result, we have to maintain a certain vigilance about minimizing our exposure. If you want to have the best chance at resisting the effects of environmental toxicity, however, you need to start with a "clean slate." That means detoxifying from whatever metals and other toxins you have inevitably accumulated over the years.

As we discussed earlier, mercury is one of the most prevalent internal toxic heavy metals. It accumulates gradually in the fatty tissues—including the brain. Yet many health practitioners are not trained to look into the mouth when treating syndromes such as lupus, autism, CFS, fibromyalgia, and multiple sclerosis, yet most all of them are traceable to some form of heavy metal toxicity.

Getting a proper diagnosis for this kind of toxicity is made more difficult by the views of the key medical organizations. The American Dental Association, for instance, maintains there is no correlation between poor health and mercury. I believe that's a little like saying there is no correlation between low-hanging dark clouds and rain. Recently, though, the FDA's dental research arm, the National Institute of Dental Research, has made baby steps into researching the subject. In the meantime, it's worthwhile to remember the maxim that: "Absence of proof is not proof of absence."

Suspecting the connection between heavy metal toxicity and poor health is reasonable. There is enough informal evidence and anecdotal positive results from treatment that it makes sense to take appropriate action to reduce our toxicity levels.

Mercury and Other Toxic Conspirators

The primary culprits in causing toxin buildup are stress, the physical environment, the standard American diet, and heavy metals, including many cosmetics and almost all medications. Mercury, lead, cadmium, arsenic, pesticides, insecticides, vaccines, dioxins, furans, phthalates, volatile organic compounds (found in many environmental pollutants), and PCBs are just some of the toxic substances that have created toxic body burdens in our daily living. But "public enemy #1" in the world of internal toxins is mercury.

Mercury exists in three different forms:

- **Elemental Mercury, HG.** This mercury has no electrical charge and is the kind contained in mercury fillings. It has the most deleterious effect on the brain, immune system, and reproductive system.
- **Ionic Mercury, HG++.** This mercury is positively charged and is readily absorbed in the gut. Its primary negative effects occur in the cellular membrane and the digestive system. It also causes autoimmune dysfunction.
- **Methyl Mercury, CH3HG++.** This is the mercury vapor form and can be deadly to ingest. Methyl mercury affects the lungs, eyes, and uterus, and causes neurological damage.[*]

Because of traditional dentistry methodologies, most of us have been subjected to elemental mercury through the implantation of silver fillings, every one of which contains anywhere from 43 to 55 percent pure elemental mercury. The release of mercury into the body begins immediately upon placing the filling in the mouth and continues through the life of the filling by emitting mercury vapors. The presence of ten average amalgam fillings in the mouth amounts to about five grams of mercury, which continuously leak mercury vapor. This is especially troubling in vapor form since it has been documented that inhaled mercury vapor has an 80 percent absorption rate.[†]

Once in the body, mercury has a frightening track record. Mercury toxicity shuts down production of hydrochloric acid in the stomach, causing digestive problems. It also increases autoimmune dysfunction and inhibits normal thyroid functioning. In pregnant women, heavy metals like mercury can cross the placental barrier and end up in the blood of the umbilical cord. The troubling presence of mercury is confirmed through autopsies which show that the number of amalgam fillings in the mouth correlates with the amount of mercury found in brain tissue, in kidneys, and in the pituitary, thyroid, and adrenal glands.[‡]

This is all because chronic exposure (i.e., ongoing exposure such as that produced by the presence of mercury fillings) to even minute doses of mercury causes an accumulation of mercury over the lifetime of the affected organism. Accumulation occurs because the body has a difficult time eliminating mercury without specific help in doing so.

---

* IAOMT, http://www.iaomt.org.

† IAOMT, *Smoking Teeth*, video, https://toothbody.com/smoking-teeth/.

‡ IAOMT, Conference lecture notes, 2018.

These are many of the problems that can be attributed to heavy metal toxicity, of which mercury is the worst offender:

- Decreased thyroid function.
- Decreased gut function and reduced HCL production in the stomach, caused by a corresponding increase in stomach Hg-Cl, which is toxic.
- Decreased nitric oxide (NO) and endothelial function (NO is the "molecule of life" that supports healthy cell and vascular function.
- Neurological diseases including autistic spectrum disorders.
- Interferes with ATP energy production by displacing magnesium.
- Inactivates critical enzyme systems.
- Crosses the placental membrane and is absorbed by the fetus.
- Likely connected to Alzheimer's disease.
- Linked to some instances of the most extreme cases of high blood pressure.
- Alters ribosomal DNA synthesis of protein.
- Contributes to leaky gut and leaky (blood) vessel syndromes.
- Contributes to high blood pressure.*

Daily attention to diet, lifestyle, and your immediate environment, plus a nutritional regimen that supports the liver conjugation (conversion of waste substances for removal) and excretion of bodily toxins is paramount. The release of your stored body toxins, though, must be accompanied by a plan for safely ejecting them from the body. Otherwise, toxic waste can build up and cause extreme sickness.†

The Oral Rejuvenation, Heavy Metal Detoxification Plan

Because heavy metal toxicity is so underdiagnosed, you may not receive much support from a traditional practitioner if you decide to detoxify. But don't let any doctor or dentist tell you it's not important. In fact, the way you do it is as critical as making sure that you do it—especially when it involves removal of mercury fillings.

Safe mercury removal is absolutely critical because the release of mercury vapor increases exponentially during this process, and since mercury vapor combines readily with fatty tissues, it can affect every cell membrane of every one of your 70 or so trillion cells—including those in your brain.

When mercury vapor is released, it binds to sulfur, which is the by-product of bacterial activity (i.e., infection), and it becomes methylated mercury. This is the deadlier form and is the primary reason you need someone trained in proper

---

* Thomas E. Levy, MD, JD, *Hidden Epidemic* (MedFox Publishing, 2017) 67–68.

† Budapest Study.

mercury-removal techniques. So, filling removal is the starting point. Otherwise, you can do a full-body cleanse, only to have mercury rereleased into your system through your fillings.

Before you start the detox protocol, there are some preparatory steps you need to take in order to prepare your body for the release and elimination of toxins. Your body, after all, has been sequestering these toxins in an effort to keep you safe from them, but when you pull them out of hiding, the body has to manage them, and that can be difficult. You must have a healthy immune system to handle what is to come during the seven to twelve months detoxification will require.

So, assuming you've gotten rid of your amalgam fillings and are ready to start the detoxification process in earnest, what do you do to prepare for the rest of the process? To begin with, you must make sure your colon is functioning properly. This is critical: Do not start any detoxification protocol if you are constipated. If you are not eliminating everyday, then you need to do a colon cleanse before you proceed with any other detoxification.

These are the supplements, therapies, and available sources for colon cleansing:

1. Aqueous magnesium chloride (caution: can cause explosive diarrhea)
2. Global Healing Colon Cleanse
3. Ballerina tea or senna tea
4. B-Sure Colon Health (100 percent psyllium husk powder)
5. Colonics by a qualified hydro-colon therapist
6. Complete Cleansing Fiber, Part 2 (from Trace Minerals Research)
7. Organic Bowel Cleanse (from Renew Life)
8. Cascara sagrada, "aged bark" (425 mg is a stimulant laxative)
9. Metabolic Cleanse (from Douglas Laboratories)
10. Metabolic Rejuvenation (from Douglas Laboratories).

After you've unclogged your drain, you're ready to work on other vital organs in the detox process. I recommend going through a formal liver and gall bladder cleanse.

Here's how.*

- **Follow a strict anti-inflammatory diet for one month.** This includes following the Dirty Dozen and Clean 15 guidelines (Appendix). You'll want to achieve an 80/20 alkaline diet by making sure 80 percent of your foods are alkaline.

* Biotics Research, http://www.bioticsresearch.com/research-and-education.

- **Take one of these for three months: Paleocleanse, Biotics Nutriclear, or Pro Toxi-Clear.**
- **Consume one fresh-squeezed lemon**, three times a day, in a tall glass of clean water, to alkalinize your system and the biofilm in your mouth.
- **Take ground flaxseed**—two heaping tablespoons in the morning and at night.
- **Massage to increase lymphatic drainage**. You can do this yourself with Vibrational Power Plate usage twice a day.
- **Walk a minimum of twenty minutes per day** or 10,000 steps (monitor with a Fitbit).
- **Take chlorophyll** in the morning and at night.
- **Use Green Powder. Use only olive oil and coconut oil for cooking and salads** (but don't overheat your oil when cooking). Stay far away from store-bought dressings.
- **Take Argentyn 23**, professional-grade silver hydrosol to eliminate all oral and GI infections. It's also a great natural antibiotic with healing properties. (Also, add Sovereign Copper).
- **Take oregano** (excellent for eliminating GI parasites).
- **Limit your consumption of potatoes and bananas** since they are high-glycemic foods.
- **Avoid all processed foods**—especially sugar.
- **Eat fresh ginger and pineapple** daily.
- **Eat only organic fruits and vegetables** that are in season.
- **Take chlorella** in the morning and at night.
- **Take spirulina** every morning.
- **Eat one clove of aged garlic** every day.
- **Take R-Lipoic acid** (600 mg).
- **Eat a lot of arugula.**
- **Eat beets, beets, and more beets.**
- **Take Liposomal glutathione (500mg) or a Meyers Cocktail I-V. Take Dim or Indole-3-Carbinol.** This is fantastic for lowering estrone levels and reducing PSA levels in men.
- **Use Mega Green Tea with Green Coffee Extract** (absorbs 60 percent better than regular green tea).
- **Use N-Acetyl Cysteine,** also called NAC (can use as a nasal inhalant), synthesized from methionine and serine (especially important to take this after mercury removal).
- **Take L-arginine** (if you're over 40, take the NEO-40 version).
- **Take calcium-D glucarate** (500 mg daily).
- **Pearl Nature's Toothpaste®** (boosts salivary nitric oxide).

In addition, if you want to ramp up your detoxification preparation, there are a few other "nice to have" things you can do. An ion cleanse, for instance, is a type of footbath that detoxifies through the bottom of your feet. It is likewise helpful to increase your overall consumption of fiber, and if you feel that handling stress is a particular issue for you, seeing a counselor to help you emotionally de-stress can actually facilitate your physical detoxification. Detoxification strategies tailored for individuals with autism include infrared sauna treatments and hyperbaric oxygen therapy (HBOT). If extreme fatigue or fibromyalgia are among your issues, you might want to consider HBOT and D-ribose.

The Importance of Safe Mercury Amalgam Removal

The purpose of removing mercury amalgam from your teeth is to eliminate a major source of heavy metal toxicity and thus, prevent inflammation from entering your body's biosystem. However, the removal of mercury amalgam is potentially extremely dangerous to you, me, and our staff. It is also dangerous to the environment if certain proven safety measures are not followed. The IAOMT and IABDM protocols that we use include most, if not all, of the following:*

- Supplements to include cleansing foods that you can begin any time prior to your appointment.
- A watertight rubber dam barrier, flossed around the necks of the teeth.
- A saliva ejector placed under the barrier to remove mercury vapor.
- A high-speed suction placed next to the operating field, called an Isolite.
- Rather than drilling the mercury indiscriminately, we section and remove the filling in chunks.
- A high-volume Dent-Air-Vacuum placed next to your chin (elephant trunk).
- A negative ion generator placed in the office to bind up any mercury vapor that escapes the vacuums.
- Copious amounts of water sprayed at the amalgam to keep it cool.
- Available medical oxygen delivered through a N2O monitoring system mask.
- A mercury trap (mercury separator) in place that contains 100 percent of the mercury waste.

These steps are taken to provide your body with the least amount of mercury exposure possible, thus allowing the best possible chance of an improvement to your health.

* IAOMT, *Smoking Teeth*, video, https://toothbody.com/smoking-teeth/.

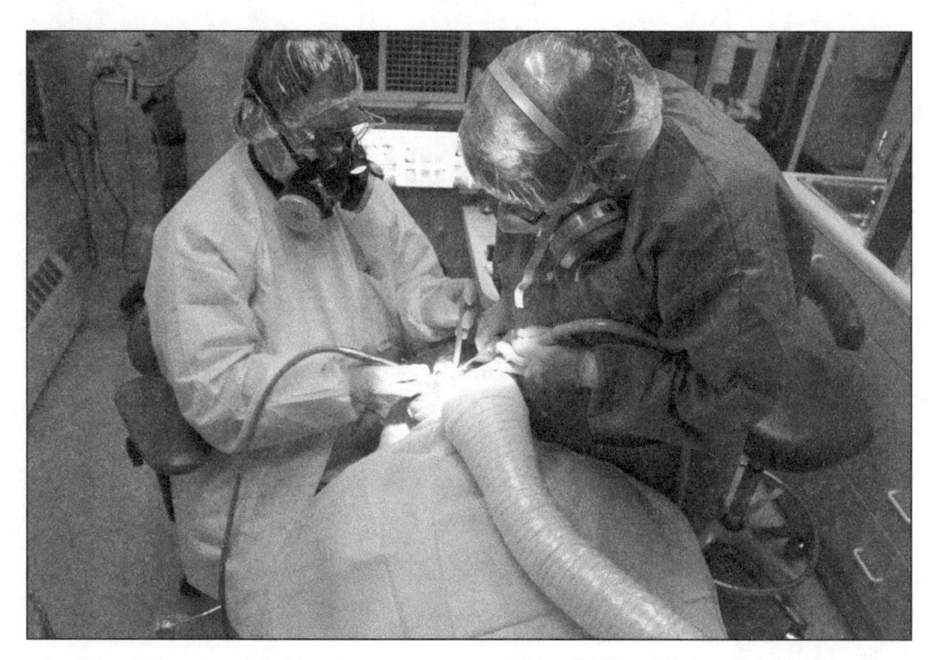

Amalgam filling removal procedure with protection from mercury vapor and particles. Credit: Tribune Content Agency LLC.

The Special Role of Glutathione in Detoxification

Glutathione in the reduced form, called GSH, is a helpful body chemical that greatly aids in the detoxification process, but it must be "coddled" a bit to make sure it works well for you. The process by which it works is to donate electrons to bind with free radicals (to neutralize them) and to produce energy in the metabolism cycle. In its oxidized form, though, GSSG glutathione is not as helpful. Some is necessary, but it must be in a much lesser quantity than the GSH, or reduced form.

GSH is your body's most potent antioxidant because it helps to maintain a high redox potential, the opportunity to "absorb" extra electrons (free radicals) in the blood system. In fact, low levels of GSH have been known to cause death in elderly people. In addition, low levels of glutathione have been found to contribute to neurological diseases such as Parkinson's, autism, and Alzheimer's disease. And, low GSH can cause fatigue, muscle aches, and mood swings. It has also been linked to diabetes.* For our purposes, healthy GSH levels are necessary for immune functioning. As your body detoxifies, GSH becomes critical to the "mopping-up" operation whereby free radicals are eliminated.

* Thomas J. Lewis, PhD, and Clement L. Trempe, MD. *The End of Alzheimer's; The Brain and Beyond* (2014).

The Importance of Chelation Therapy

Chelation therapy has been proven in thousands of clinical examples to effectively remove toxic metals from the body. In fact, according to the infamous CDC, more than 60,000 Americans have used some form of chelation therapy in the past twelve years, and many major health insurers such as Aetna, Blue Cross, and Cigna now have policies endorsing chelation therapy as the appropriate way to address heavy metal toxicity, including vaccine injuries.

Chelation is the process of removing toxic metals from your body's biosystem. Toxic metals are the most difficult to remove from the tissues, and in the process, other nontoxic beneficial minerals may be removed as well. To minimize this downside, care and skill are required so that essential macro- and micronutrients are not depleted. The "upside" of chelation, though, makes it worth the risks that can be minimized with proper implementation of the protocol. As outlined below, chelation benefits the body in almost every way.

Here's how:

Heart and Blood Vessels[*, †]

- Helps prevent arteriosclerosis (hardening of the arteries) by removing calcium with EDTA.
- Rejuvenates your cardiovascular system by increasing ENOS, the enzyme that boosts NO.
- Improves conduction in all degrees of A-V heart block.
- Helps abolish extra heartbeats, skipped beats, and rapid heartbeats.
- Decreases ventricular arrhythmia due to digitalis toxicity.
- Reduces blood pressure and blood cholesterol.
- Improves circulation by increasing nitric oxide.[‡, §]
- Reduces varicose veins.
- Reduces stroke and heart attack aftereffects.
- Reduces heart irritability.
- Reduces heart valve calcification.
- Makes arterial walls more flexible.
- Reduces excessive heart contractions.
- Dissolves fat deposits in plaque-lined arteries.
- Prevents LDL cholesterol deposits.

---

* IAOMT, Conference lecture notes, 2018.

† A4M, 17th Annual World Congress on Anti-Aging & Regenerative Medicine Conference (San Jose, CA, Sept 9–12, 2009).

‡ Laird, et al., https://rumble.com/v31sisg-nitric-oxide-the-miracle-molecule.html.

§ http://www.CardioMiracle.com.

Brain and Nervous System

- Reduces Alzheimer's disease-like symptoms.
- Helps to relieve symptoms of senility by increasing circulation to the brain.
- Helps to relieve pain and reduces hypoglycemia, phlebitis, and scleroderma.
- Improves memory.
- Helps make blood slippery and prevents abnormal blood clotting.

Eyes, Kidney, Liver, and Other Organs

- Improves vision and hearing.
- Improves skin texture and tone.
- Dissolves kidney stones.
- Dissolves small cataracts.
- Decreases macular degeneration.
- Improves liver function.
- Improves vision in diabetic retinopathy.
- Heals calcified necrotic ulcers.

Disease Prevention and Healing

- Reverses diabetic gangrene.
- Reduces rheumatoid arthritis symptoms.
- Lowers diabetics' insulin needs.
- Detoxifies snake and spider venoms.
- Helps as a preoperative preparation.
- Prevents osteoarthritis.
- Reduces intermittent claudication (leg cramping).

You may have heard that chelation therapy is not entirely safe. I can assure you, though, that when handled properly, any danger is minimal. The side effects of chelation at the dosing levels used with children appear to be both mild and manageable. The mineral depletion I mentioned earlier is the most obvious negative side effect, but it can be managed through mineral repletion by supplementing with minerals. One very straightforward recommendation is simply to use Concentrace® Trace Mineral Drops (twenty-one to thirty-four drops per day to bowel tolerance), along with the addition of six to ten Pearl Silica Drops®.

A secondary potential side effect is kidney or liver stress induced by the pace of detoxification. This is addressed by temporarily adjusting the dosage. Most doctors treating autistic children run monthly or bimonthly lab tests to monitor for these issues, but even this downside is totally manageable under the right supervision. Consult an integrative or functional specialist.

The four principal methods for chelation are oral, intravenous, dermal, and rectal. These are some excellent chelation products:

- Lipo-Phos EDTA, from Allergy Research Group
- I-V DMSO or DMSA
- Iodoral, 32.5 milligrams, not micrograms
- Polyamino, poly-carbonic acid, and disodium EDTA
- Hyper-Oxy-Ozone Suppositories
- B-vitamins, which vastly increase endothelial function and the production of NO, NAD+
- NCD, Natural Cellular Defense (15 ml daily), a powdered form of zeolite
- Clinoptilolite (24 mg daily)
- Detoxamin, rectal suppositories for kids and adults
- Livaplex, a natural antibiotic that digests bacteria
- Results RNA, a zeolite
- Advanced TRS, a zeolite from COSEVA
- Global Healing: Heavy Metal & Chemical Cleaner
- Quick-Silver Scientific, IMD and an array of products

How Your Body Detoxifies

Your skin is the largest detoxification exit portal in your body. Especially if other, inner pathways are restricted, the skin will attempt to expel toxic cellular waste. This can be in the form of a rash, boils, other skin eruptions, or sweating (the preferable way). Because perspiration is a good conductor of toxins, using an infrared sauna can help greatly in detoxing.

The body also expels toxins through the lungs via blood gases (CO_2 and other toxic gases). Chinese practitioners, in fact, are so well aware of the breath's role dispersing toxins that smelling a patient's breath is part of their diagnostic exam. If odor from the mouth is not caused by microbial breakdown on the tongue or around teeth—as in typical halitosis—it is from blood gases. These gases can be released from microbial breakdown or from the breakdown of toxic residues. To use a familiar example of the same process in other forms: underarm odor is the oxidation and breakdown of microbial activity.

The colon route of elimination is another extremely important avenue of detoxification. Your intestine is designed for eliminating large molecular, toxic, and microbial debris. After food is broken down and the good nutrients absorbed through the wall of the small intestine, the residue or undigested debris goes into the large intestine. By analogy, it's helpful to think of the large intestine as a trash compactor. It compresses this debris, extracts water and any usable nutrients, and absorbs them through its membrane wall. Some toxic elements may also be absorbed back into the bloodstream if there is too much coming from the small intestine, or if the liver has not converted the toxic elements into excretable products, or if there are not enough binders in the large intestine (such as fiber and chlorella).

The colon is the last section of tube that expels waste. For the cellular waste to even get to the large intestine to be compacted and eliminated, however, the lymphatic system has to have collected the cellular waste, the lymph nodes (immune organs) have to disinfect and neutralize it, and these toxins then must be carried to the liver for detoxification conversion—all part of the detoxification process. This conversion system is called the cytochrome P-450 system, which resides in the liver.

Hence, the liver and lymphatic systems are also critical to heavy metal removal. You can think of lymph fluid as our cellular cleanup and transport system. It runs parallel to the circulatory system. Unlike the circulatory system, however, the lymphatic system is not driven by a pump. Lymphatic vessels have one-way valves to let fluid move in only one direction. These valves open and close, causing a gentle suction by which the cellular waste is drained into the lymphatic vessels. This is why you must keep moving.

Your body contains roughly 600 to 800 lymph nodes along the lymphatic vessels. These are concentrated around the organs specialized for our survival and reproduction. In the upper body, this includes the mouth, tongue, neck, breasts, and lungs. These areas in the lower regions include the colon, prostate, uterus, and ovaries as well as collection points around the hips and the top of the legs. It's not a coincidence that these are the areas where most cancers occur because lymph nodes are the immune organs that break down toxic or infective waste.

Once the lymph nodes have done their job, the lymphatic waste travels to the liver and large intestine for elimination. Then the lymph fluid is recirculated back into the venous system. So, you can see how all-encompassing the detoxification process has to be in order to function correctly.[*, †]

Do You Need to Detox?

Obviously, you want to undertake a whole-body detoxification only if you really need it. And fortunately, there is some highly reliable testing you can do to evaluate your heavy metal load. The first step I recommend is to give yourself the thirty-one-question self-assessment in Appendix 3. Your answers will determine if you're a likely candidate for further testing by a medical professional which will then help you decide how to proceed.

---

* Morton Walker, DPM, Garry Gordon, MD, DO, and W. C. Douglass, MD, *The Chelation Answer: How to Prevent Hardening of the Arteries and Rejuvenate Your Cardiovascular System* (Second Opinion Pub, Inc, 1993).

† IAOMT, *Detoxification*, https://iaomt.org/resources/.

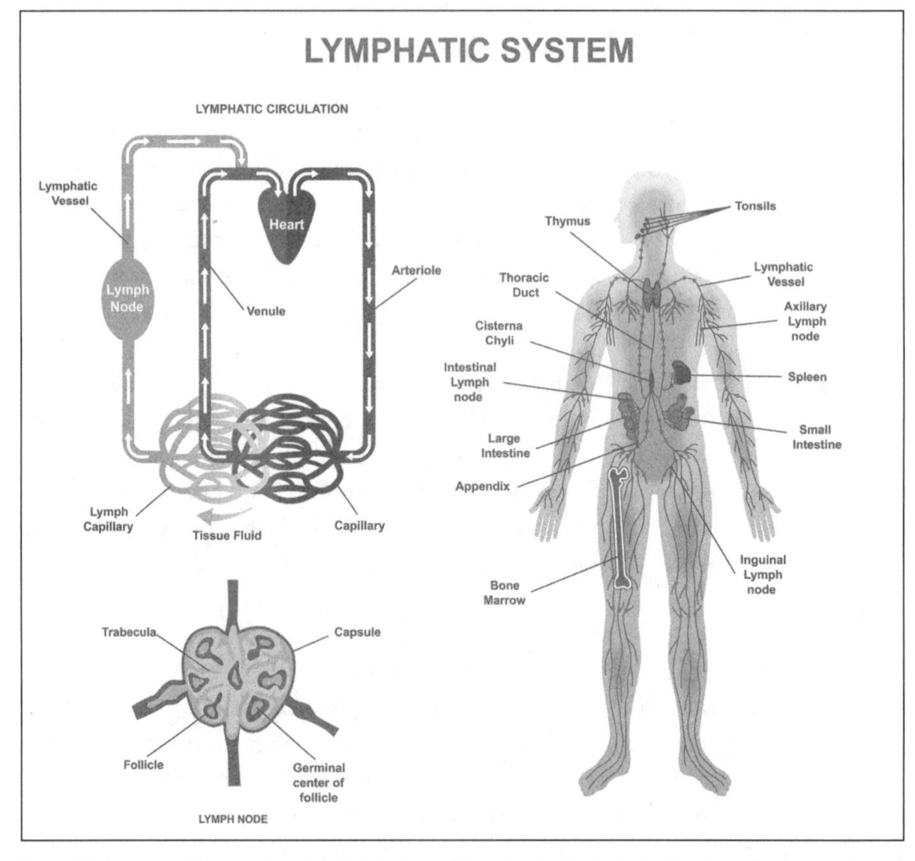

Lymphatic system illustrating the circulation of lymphatic fluid, including lymphatic vessels and nodes throughout the body. Credit: Rudzhan Nagiev.

Assuming that you discover a need for detoxing, it's helpful to know about the common next-step tests in the exploration process, so I've outlined below some testing options your physician can provide.

1. Heavy metal challenge testing (available through Doctors Data or Genova Laboratories)
2. Mercury tri-test (from Quicksilver Scientific), a blood, urine, and hair analysis
3. HMT, DMPS urinary challenge testing (from Metametrix)
4. Rita Meter testing, to evaluate the ionic charge in mercury fillings. It measures milli-voltage.
5. Spectra-cell testing, to detect nutrient deficiencies, called a Spectrox test
6. Porphyrin testing. Because urinary porphyrins are the biomarkers of toxicity that reveal toxicants in the body's critical biochemical pathways

(available from Metametrix). Increased urinary porphyrins indicate toxic levels of mercury, lead, arsenic, and other unwanted organic chemicals.

7. Ameritox, specifically to determine the presence of drug toxicity (from Medication Monitoring Solutions)

Once you've discovered your personal toxicity profile, you'll need to work with a medical professional trained in detox procedures to set up the right protocol for your situation. Before we conclude our discussion of whole-body detoxification, I'd like to say a few words about a couple of specific, common situations that necessitate a detox protocol.

Special Case #1: Detoxing for Weight Control

If you want to attain your ideal weight and improve your health in the process, you need to start with detoxification. Heavy metal toxicity can correlate strongly with weight problems.

Lead toxicity, for example, can result in unhealthy weight *loss* while mercury toxicity can result in hypothyroidism and weight *gain*. Heavy metals also interact with each other.

When both lead and mercury are present, the detrimental effects of mercury increase significantly. Heavy metal toxicity also results in digestive tract disturbances such as bloating, constipation or diarrhea, abdominal pain, nausea, and vomiting. Heavy metals accumulated in the body can cause liver damage, and since fat regulation is one of the most important functions of the liver, it will become impaired and cause you to gain weight.

Special Case #2: Detoxing for Autism Healing

Heavy metal toxicity is an especially serious problem for children. Dr. Woeller, an integrative medicine physician and biomedical autism specialist, explains:*

> Most damage occurs to the neurological system when it is forming! The research on autistic children has shown that they have the lowest levels of mercury in blood, hair, and urine analysis. These children are the most susceptible and affected by mercury. The conclusion here: is that they are not excreting or eliminating the mercury, but retaining it in the brain tissue. This explains their lower test levels. Autistic children have the lowest levels of mercury in blood and urine and hair, whereas: non-autistic children: have the highest levels of mercury in their hair, blood, and urine and are the least affected because they are excreting heavy metals. There is an inverse relationship between measurable levels of mercury and the degree of autism.

---

* Kurt N. Woeller, DO, *Autism: The Road to Recovery* (CreateSpace Independent Publishing Platform, 2012).

The connection could hardly be clearer. Heavy metal toxicity correlates directly with autism in children. This is because mercury poisons glial cells and interferes with their uptake of glutamate. As a result, the cells cannot rid the brain of stored toxins. This problem facilitates the crossing of the blood-brain barrier (BBB) by the mercury, even though the barrier is there to prevent just such an invasion of toxic material. Mercury is unleashed to decrease mitochondrial function and to destroy enzymes and production of energy-generating ATP. It also inhibits proper thyroid functioning.*

So, if you suspect your child (or yourself) of having some level of autism, you absolutely need to evaluate whether heavy metals are in play. While many people lament that autism is "incurable," you may find out that it's not. In fact, the more you delve into whole-body medicine, the more you may discover that many "incurable" diseases are not so incurable after all.

One final caution: Do not ever succumb to the barrage of vaccines that are heaped upon our innocent children or yourself without verifiable safety testing.

Vaccines are full of aluminum and mercury in the form of thimerosal and are highly toxic. †

The mRNA vaccines are not even vaccines at all.

---

* Woeller, *Autism: the Road to Recovery.*

† *Vaxxed*, https://vaxxedthemovie.com/.

PART FOUR

Key Solutions for Whole-Body Health and Antiaging Medicine

CHAPTER 15

The Whole-Health Lifestyle

Insurance treats disease from the old HMO disease model which is based on a seven-minute doctor visit to control costs. The wellness approach, however, is the exact opposite. It prevents disease by using newer antiaging testing and technologies to sustain health and identify problems before they become systemic. Because popping pills is not the answer to good health, in this chapter, I'm going to give you an overview of additional health practices you can integrate into your lifestyle to help your body operate at its very best.

Become Anti-Antibiotics and Pro-Probiotics

"In 4.5 billion years, nothing has ever developed a resistance to silver. It took only a scant seven decades for pharmaceuticals to fail across the board."*

The CEO of the Immunogenics Corporation of Florida is clear about the abysmal failure of pharmaceutical drugs. Besides damaging the body's system of good bacteria, systemic antibiotics cause unwanted yeast to flourish. On the other hand, Argentyn-23, nano-silver hydrosol, is a wholly safe and effective way to eradicate unwanted bacteria. It is also viricidal and fungicidal. You also cannot develop an immunity to A-23. Same with hypochlorous acid, which is a component of OxyMist® and naturally produced by your white blood cells. WBCs kill bacteria and viruses, even TB! The unspoken paradigm of big pharmaceutical firms is to "keep patients sick but symptom-free." That way, customers keep coming back for more medicine to suppress symptoms while root causes persist. The false promise is that you can maintain an acceptable quality of life while the body deteriorates from the profound acidic damage inflicted by modern pharmaceutical "solutions" to medical problems and the standard American diet (SAD). Oxy-Mist and Argentyn-23 belong in your health arsenal for those times when killing pathogenic bacteria, viruses, and fungus is a must. You can nebulize both.

* https://naturalimmunogenics.com/

Optimize Your Whole-Body Systems

Throughout this book, we've talked about the various systems in your body that must operate at optimal levels to make you truly healthy. Being aware of what these systems are is key to monitoring your own health and taking the initiative to be sure you're treating yourself (and being treated by practitioners) with the whole picture in mind. So, just to give you the overview in one place, here's a list of the body's systems that need to be optimized:

- The digestive, elimination and lymphatic systems
- The brain, neurotransmitter, and bioenergy systems
- The inflammatory system and control of NF-k Beta
- The blood and cardiac system, including mitochondrial support
- The glandular, hormonal system
- The muscle and skeletal systems
- The immunological system

The Immune and Chromosomal (DNA) support systems

While it's beyond the scope of this book to fully address each of these, taking the "high road" to health we've been talking about—eating right, detoxing, supplementing, et al.—will go a long way to setting you up for a healthy lifestyle. I've created a detailed program that explores in-depth the way to maximize each of these systems, and I hope when you're ready, you'll take advantage of working through the plans I've laid out. In most cases, optimizing your health in a focused program takes about a year of dedicated work, but in relation to the benefits for the rest of your life, that's not much time.

Remineralize Your Life, Teeth, and Skeletal Matrix

To achieve optimal health, you must have balanced adrenal glands because adrenal glands are the key to balancing your mineral ratios. This process maintains body balance through proper alkalization. Your adrenal function also synthesizes, from cholesterol, sex hormones, and stress neurotransmitters that you need. Junk diets cannot help you maintain proper nutrient content to keep your adrenals healthy. Eating proper nutrition and essential nutrients will keep the balance of these required elements. These are the minerals you need:

- Calcium (Ca^{++})
- Silica (Si^{+}) in the form of OSA
- Magnesium (Mg^{++})
- Sodium (Na^{+})
- Potassium (K^{+})

- Phosphorous (P+, not PO4+++—phosphate,), because increased phosphate levels decrease zinc, calcium, and magnesium and upsets your electrolytic balance.
- Boron (B)
- Molybdenum (Mo)
- Zinc (Zn++)
- Copper (Cu++) just a trace
- Selenium, about 800mcgs per day, along with:
- Iodine, *at least* 12.5 mg per day (not mcgs)
- Potassium

And here are some guidelines to keeping your minerals balanced correctly:

- **The calcium to phosphorus ratio needs to be 2.5 to 1.** This can be thrown off by the introduction of too much phosphate into your system and is why the excess of phosphate in soft drinks is so bad. The phosphate ion (PO4) in soda pop adds way too much phosphate into your body.
- **Do not take calcium with iron.** When they compete, calcium wins, and iron becomes oxidized and damages other important nutrients.
- **Lead interferes with the body's ability to use calcium** (another reason to detox).
- **Mercury is an uncoupler** and messes up enzymatic balance (detox!).
- **Keep iodine and selenium in balance**—don't high-dose either one.
- **Minimize coffee and tea consumption** because they can contain high levels of fluoride, nickel, and cadmium.
- **Keep alcohol consumption to a minimum** because it blocks selenium.
- **Eat a lot of these to maintain healthy levels of selenium:** shiitake mushrooms, eggs, garlic, broccoli, asparagus, salmon, spinach, and oats.
- **Maintain healthy zinc levels** by eating non-processed red meats (zinc is critical in making stomach acid, without which you cannot digest your food).
- **In addition to drinking pure water, eat plenty of these hydrating foods:** celery, cantaloupe, tomatoes, lettuce, pears, blueberries, grapefruit, pineapple, watermelon, cucumber.

Treat your body well in these ways, and it does a fantastic job at compensating for injury. Each organ system and each of your estimated 70 trillion cells are programmed by DNA to repair themselves. An extremely important part of this remarkable ability, the process of remineralization, is greatly enhanced by removing toxic mercury from your teeth before beginning other remineralization efforts.

Remineralization can greatly benefit your skeletal bony matrix as well as your teeth. And, of course, eliminating processed sugars from your diet is a must for remineralization.*

Tapping into your body's innate ability to heal itself, remineralization will occur naturally when you:

- Eliminate processed sugar consumption.
- Boost your nitric oxide level.†
- Use green coffee bean extract for its chlorogenic acid content.
- Increase the protein in your diet—especially hemp protein, flaxseed, chia seeds, and other branched chain amino acids, especially L-leucine. Eat these often. Mostly plant-based protein with 5 to 10 percent animal protein. Watch the *Forks over Knives* documentary.
- Eat grass-fed red meat. Consume cold-water fish with scales only. No catfish, sorry.
- Use Celtic sea salt and Concentrace® Mineral Drops‡ to augment your macro-minerals.
- Increase consumption of trace minerals and silica (Pearl Silica Drops™).§
- Take fat-soluble vitamins, especially vitamin D. Increase your consumption of raw and sautéed vegetables.
- Eat raw dairy products and cheese, kefir and yogurt made from raw dairy—not the kind you can get in stores. Supplement with zinc, selenium, and magnesium.
- Take physician-grade prebiotics along with your probiotics.¶
- Eat more fermented foods; these are great for probiotic content.
- Use Ancient Nutrition SBO probiotics.
- Eat plenty of healthy fats, including some saturated fats.
- Eat eggs, especially the yolks, raw or soft boiled; they are a good source of choline for improved memory function.
- Get at least twenty minutes of sunshine per day—before 11:00 a.m. or after 2:30 p.m. (do not use sunscreen).
- Eat only foods that are in season and vine-ripened.
- Use bone broth (I use Ancient Nutrition).
- Eat pumpkin seeds, dates, almonds, and Brazil nuts (best to soak almonds first).

---

* Lokensgard, Patients Guide to Remineralization of Teeth and Bone, Protocol, http://www.drlokensgard.com/shop.

† https://cardiomiracle.com/.

‡ http://www.traceminerals.com.

§ http://www.PearlOralHealth.com.

¶ Laird Wellness Live, https://rumble.com/v4nmaqh-enzymes-who-what-when-where-why-how.html.

- Use colostrum (best from New Zealand).
- Use cod liver oil (I use Dr. Stephen Sinatra's regimen, esp., Omega Plus 100 with Resveratrol).
- Avoid prescription medicines as much as possible, especially stomach acid blockers.
- Stop eating processed food, especially processed animal foods as it raises the hormone IGF-1.

For those of you who need a quick refresher on, "Hey, just tell me what to do!": This is what to do, on a daily basis. First, familiarize yourself with my Remineralization Protocol*:

- Balance your mineral content with Concentrace® Mineral Drops and Pearl Silica Drops®.
- Use Cardio Miracle® to boost nitric oxide.†
- Use homemade bone broth or Bone Broth Protein powders from Ancient Nutrition.‡
- Use our Pearl Nature's Toothpaste®. Kids love it too.
- Eat an 80 percent alkaline diet (see the list in the Appendix).
- Eat more fermented foods.
- Alkalinize your oral flora by rinsing with Bob's Red Meal Baking Soda.
- Follow the safe sugars, but use xylitol sparingly.
- Follow the recommended anti-inflammatory foods list.
- One option is to use fermented cod-liver oil.
- Use ghee, coconut oil, and grass-fed butter.
- Follow a Weston A. Price diet with raw milk.
- Consider the Forks over Knives diet.
- Consider not eating pork.
- Consider a keto diet with high-quality fats, moderate protein, and very low carbohydrates.
- Include humic and fulvic acid in your nutrient supplementation protocol.
- Essential oils can also be extremely helpful.

The Special Case of Breastfeeding

The benefits of breastfeeding versus formula-feeding can hardly be overstated. This is the starting point for a healthy immune system and proper facial development. If your baby starts out this way, the benefits will last a lifetime.

---

* Dr. Thomas Lokensgard, Patients Guide to Remineralization of Teeth and Bone, Protocol, http://www.drlokensgard.com/shop.

† https://cardiomiracle.com/.

‡ AncientNutrition.com.

Breastfeeding is extremely beneficial for the developing infant. As a child develops during the first two years of life, the immune system is "under construction." It's a key time to make sure your child gets the God-given nutrients he or she needs. Breast milk provides all of the essential nutrients. By contrast, if you look at labels on the most popular infant formulas, you'll see that they are full of synthetic sugars and fillers. It's a travesty that the Food and Drug Administration endorses this stuff.

For the first three months, breastfeeding provides these benefits to mother and child:

- The mother's antibodies
- Healthy proteins
- Healthy fats
- Increased oxytocin (the bonding hormone)
- Decreased postpartum depression
- Increased brain function
- Colostrum
- Increased immune system support
- Decreased respiratory infections
- Less overall infections and colic
- Decreased chance of breast cancer in women
- Decreased incidence of colitis later in life
- Helps to develop lower jaw and lower face, palate and airway space.

So, if you're still in your child-bearing years, do your babies an incredibly huge favor and breastfeed them if you possibly can.

And for yourself, remineralize, remineralize, remineralize. Your bones, teeth, and joints will thank you for it. Also take iodine 12.5 mg daily, at least, and PQQ 20 mg for a really smart baby![*]

DENTAL MERIDIANS

You've heard me say, "it's all connected," right? Well, consider that each one of your teeth corresponds to a bioelectrical acupuncture meridian. These meridians are composed of bundles of interstitial fascia that serve as one-way voltage roadways that connect your organs. Helen Langevin, MD, is a research professor of neurology at the University of Vermont. She has done a lot of work on fascial tissues, meridians, and voltage.[†, ‡]

---

* Weston A. Price Foundation; *WAPF Journal* (Fall 2017).

† *Anatomical Record* 269, no. 6 (2002): 257–65. Helen Langevin, MD, "Relationship of acupuncture points and meridians to connective tissue planes," https://onlinelibrary.wiley.com/doi/10.1002/ar.10185.

‡ Tennant, *Healing Is Voltage.*

Acupuncture meridians traditionally are believed to represent channels connecting the surface of the body to the internal organs. Think of your teeth as if they were tiny batteries lined up, each on an acupuncture circuit and when they (your teeth) become infected they shut off the power (voltage) to that circuit. Think of them as a string of lights.

This is one of the well-documented tenets of traditional Chinese medicine (TCM).*

Remember that fascial planes are made up of fibrous tissue, and this collagen tissue has the least resistance to the flow of electrons throughout the body. These tissues act as electronic semiconductors or circuits and are connected to your organs.

See the meridian tooth chart in the appendix and refer to it if you are having trouble with a specific tooth or organ system. I've found it quite useful in my daily practice. Many teeth have been drilled, filled, or crowned mistakenly, because there was an organ system failure on a meridian that was not identified. This is precisely why you need to seek the services of a biological dentistry office.

---

* The Truth About Cancer (TTAC) and The Quest for the Cures; Bollinger, Ty and Charlene; Convention and Video Series; *Eastern Medicine; Journey through Asia*, 2018. https://thetruthaboutcancer.com/category/videos/.

CHAPTER 16

A Final Look at Your Teeth

Dr. Weston A. Price discovered that in all healthy societies, people eating a traditional diet for their respective areas of the world regularly manifested strong teeth and bones. Diets generally included some animal fats and plants, offering proper vitamin and mineral content. As you might guess, the good health of these people showed in their mouths. Their arches were properly developed, and their teeth were straight. This is not the case when nutrition is off-base for whatever reason—lack of food entirely or the presence of the wrong foods (a.k.a. the standard American diet).

The Importance of Fixing Crooked Teeth the Right Way

If a child is lacking in proper growth for any reason, full facial development can still be accomplished by correcting the face's bony structures using functional orthopedic correctors as early as possible in a child's developmental phase. Several factors interact to make it important to orchestrate the arranging of teeth in the optimal way.

Proper tongue position (resting on the palatal rugae) is instrumental in developing dental arches. Arches are developed by both the tongue and the associated muscles. Ties of the tongue or lip must also be identified. Dental expansion appliances then serve to put the child's tongue in the correct position and to manage the growth plates as they form the width and length of the arch. Proceeding straight to braces when palate expansion is needed causes serious negative relapse when teeth are moved improperly.

The importance of this initial step is too often overlooked because, even without managing the palate, an orthodontist can produce attractive, straight-looking teeth. The shortcut solution to crowding in the mouth is tooth removal, but unfortunately, the long-term prospects for this traditional bicuspid extraction four-on-the-floor approach to orthodontics is not so pretty.

It generally exacerbates the problem of TMJ dysfunction and provides significantly less stability for the repositioned teeth and contributes to airway obstruction.

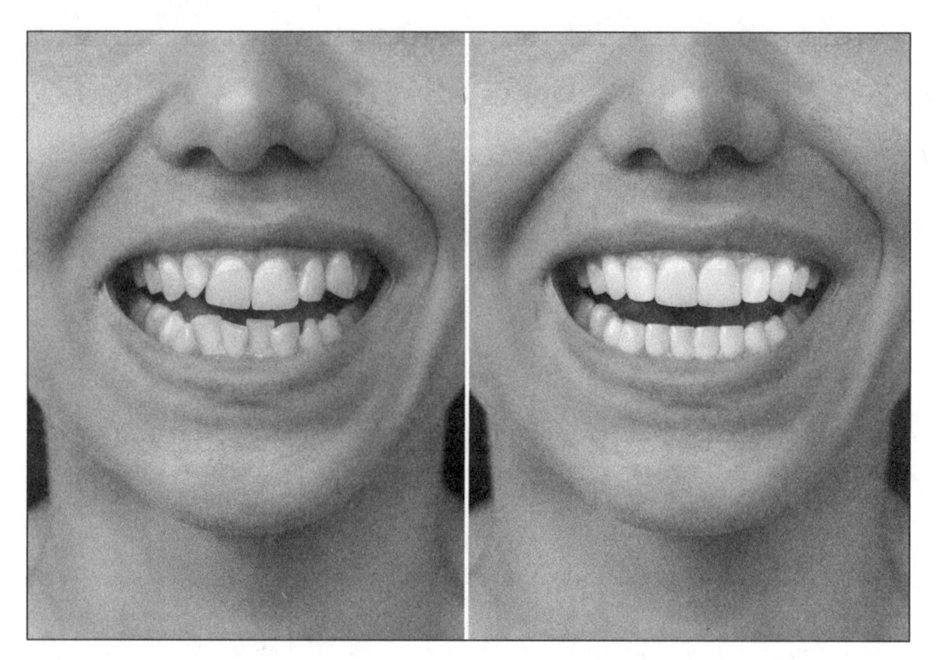

Crooked vs. straight teeth. Credit: Marina Demeshko.

If the dental arches in both upper and lower jaws are not corrected before facial growth is completed, they will remain constricted or underdeveloped. Thus, the upper and lower jaws will not have enough space to accommodate all of the permanent teeth and proper oxygenation while breathing. That's why palatal expansion (not tooth extraction) is so valuable. Braces alone do not address the underlying causes of restricted facial development and improper arch form. Timing of the procedures is also important.

When treatment is instituted early, for instance, nearly 100 percent of the malocclusions (bad bites) can be treated and improved with orthopedic expansion appliances and the remaining cases treated with straight wire appliances (fixed braces). Once a child's body has completed its growth phase, by about age eighteen, correcting the narrow bony structures in the face is much more difficult, but it can still be done, it just takes longer.

Still, there is some good news. With good nutrition and proper orthopedic expansion therapy, even after the growth phase, it is still possible to improve the facial structures as they continue to grow and thereby achieve full facial development.*

Late addressing of the problem is still far better than not addressing it at all. No matter when action is taken, braces can make the situation worse if the palate

* American Academy of Functional Orthodontics, (AAFO), Functional Orthodontics versus Traditional Orthodontics, http://www.aafo.org/.

is not managed correctly. A dysfunctional palate can leave a person with this array of unwanted problems:*

- Underdeveloped dental arches (upper and lower jaws)
- Underdeveloped sinuses and narrow nasal passages
- Constricted ear canals and constricted pituitary and pineal glands in the head
- Poor speech patterns and limited space for the tongue, tongue-ties
- Dental cross-bites
- TMJ clicking and popping
- A predisposition toward obstructive sleep apnea (OSA)
- Stage 3 to 4 tonsillar constriction
- Malocclusion (a bad bite)
- A longer-looking face, bigger-looking nose, and flatter lip profile
- Poor oral hygiene, including increased dental decay
- Posteriorly displaced condyles, which causes a retrusion of the chin
- Headaches
- Deep bites and crowded teeth
- Airway constriction, therefore less oxygen consumption and decreased ATP production via metabolism
- Less salivary and sinus output of nitric oxide levels

On the other hand, the two-phase treatment—palate first, then teeth—demonstrates a 95 percent success rate in solving the aforementioned mixed dentition issues, and this track record is accomplished without tooth extraction or surgery. Results like this can be expected, yet, the even better news is the self-esteem factor—due to improved looks and the feeling of good health—will improve as well. How about that? Good dentistry is also good psychology.

The Big Takeaways

We've covered a lot of detail in this book because the nature of functional dentistry and integrative medicine is that many different aspects of bodily health are crucial to truly good health. And admittedly, keeping track of all the details is difficult unless you're a professional looking at all of these aspects of health every day. There are, though, a few bottom lines that I hope you'll remember even if some of the "fine print" eludes you.

---

* Weston A. Price, DDS, *Nutrition and Physical Degeneration, 1939* (Price-Pottenger Nutrition Foundation Publishing, 2008).

Bottom Line #1

Good oral health is linked to healthy cardiovascular function, blood sugar metabolism and even cognitive health.

Bottom Line #2

Managing inflammation throughout the body is crucial to your well-being.

Bottom Line #3

The periodontal-related (i.e., the mouth) inflammatory response affects other parts of the body including the heart, brain, liver, and kidneys, and blood sugar metabolism, in turn, affects periodontal health.

Bottom Line #4

Silent inflammation is the root cause of chronic degenerative disease, and it starts in your mouth.

Bottom Line #5

Eliminating heavy metal toxicity is a must for good health.

Focus on addressing these items in managing your personal health and well-being, and you will set yourself up for a quality of life worth the effort you put into it.

CHAPTER 17

What About Dentistry and Cancer?

All of us have cancer cells in our bodies, but not all of us will develop cancer.
—David Servan-Schreiber, MD, PhD

The very best compilation of cancer information and interviews concerning cancer available today is, without question, the series *The Truth About Cancer* by Ty and Charlene Bollinger.* I'd highly recommend you purchase the entire series. You'll be glad you did. They have done an amazing job of gathering the expert opinions of world cancer researchers and physiological practitioners and making the information available, worldwide.

If we want to eliminate, stop, or slow down a clinical disease, condition, or infection, I have a very novel solution. How about attacking its source? The one treatment modality or element we consistently use in our office is ozone therapy (OT). We use OT to disinfect surfaces, reduce dental decay, reduce infections, reduce inflammation, and treat failed root canals as well as osteo-cavitations and periodontal disease.

The one element that attacks cancer at its source is oxygen. Ozone is like oxygen on steroids and when used correctly it raises voltage, remember? Consider for a moment that you are physiologically designed to run on oxygen with each and every breath. Oxygen is the basic fuel for your body's cellular metabolism. Remember our discussion of ATP? This is the body's fueling source and without it, you die, plain and simple.

Ozone induces healing by nontoxic wound cleansing. It kills bacteria, viruses, fungi or yeast, parasites, and almost everything that is pathogenic by creating an oxidative burst. Ozone also opens up the vascular beds by increasing NO production. It also increases production of red blood cells (RBCs), donates electrons to the Krebs cycle, and kills cancer cells by causing cellular apoptosis, thus shutting down the glycolytic pathway.

* The Truth About Cancer (TTAC) and The Quest for the Cures; Bollinger, Ty and Charlene; Convention and Video Series, https://thetruthaboutcancer.com/category/videos/.

Interestingly, human antibodies produce ozone and peroxides which are the basis of the immune system. WBCs produce HOCl, which is the same compound that is in our OxyMist®. It's a peroxide compound. These ozone breakdown products are also in human breast milk and raw cow's milk.

In his "Confidential Cures" letter, Dr. Al Sears writes: "For more than 70 years we've been told the only way to stop cancer is to wage an all-out war and that cancer cells can only be killed with toxic chemotherapy and burning radiation. Even while these so-called 'therapies' are proven to damage your brain, heart, lungs, intestines, eyes, and even your peripheral nerves." But the thing is, we've known the solution for over ninety years as more than 45,000 physicians in every country use oxygen therapies as a solution to kill all types of cancer. Even Dr. James Watson of Watson and Crick, who discovered the DNA molecule, and after nearly sixty years of advancing the "genetics causes cancer" model, has said: "We now know the current approach is not working, because on the whole, it has made no dent in cancer mortality."*

There are many other treatment modalities that work alongside or in addition to ozone therapy, some of which are suggested below. Remember: biological or physiological medicine and dentistry are focused on solving the root cause of whatever the issues are. This is why so many laypeople, moms, patients, and even doctors are getting off the polypharmacy medical-dental merry-go-round. They are taking the health of their families into their own hands.

The causes of nongenetic cancers are multimodal and the causes can be many, including a combination of:

1. Cellular O_2 deprivation (a lack of viable oxygen) contributing to voltage loss
2. Viruses, fungus (yeast), and parasites
3. Heavy metal toxicity (HMT) and dental infections, especially failed root canals
4. Emotional issues and hormonal imbalances
5. Metabolic acidosis and energy deficits
6. Environmental toxicity, including the controversial mRNA
7. Nutritional and mineral depletion

So, in treating cancer, we need to test, measure, and address all of these issues at once. Then treat with many, if not all, of the treatment modalities listed below. Please note: This list is nowhere near complete. Its purpose is to give you a starting point and a direction to go with your chosen healthcare provider.

---

* Al Sears, MD, *Confidential Cures Newsletter* (Spring 2008), 1–2.

For those of you who are having a difficult time moving away from the genetic-link theory (the belief that most cancers are genetically induced) I have good news for you.

Although symptom-based Big Pharma medicine wants you to believe that you've inherited your cancer, the truth is about 90 percent of all cancers are induced or triggered by lifestyle and nutritional deficiencies, including the biological terrain we discussed earlier. Thus, by changing your lifestyle and nutritional habits we can either slow cancer growth down or stop it altogether.*

- No mammograms, as they can cause stealth cancers; use thermographic imaging instead.
- Low levels of selenium, vitamin D3, and iodine also contribute to cancer.

You must take selenium and balance selenium with iodine. The Life Extension foundation has just completed a study that shows lowered selenium levels being related to all types of cancers. The same can be said for iodine deficiencies and vitamin D3 deficiencies, which have been well-documented.†

- Arsenic and mercury bind to selenium, this is bad news and is why you need to detoxify.
- Selenium is antineoplastic.
- Mercury and arsenic lower the bioavailability of selenium and iodine levels.
- Iodine can solubilize mercury.
- Selenium decreases double-stranded breaks in cancer genes.
- The amount of selenium to be taken daily is 800 μg.
- Do not high-dose selenium or iodine.
- BRCA-1, breast cancer carriers, are sensitive to oxidative stress.

You must also up your game when it comes to mineral content and balance, because minerals are essential for cellular membrane voltage, which controls oxygen use, which controls metabolism, which in turn makes ATP, which keeps you disease-free. I want you to memorize and be able to recite that statement to your friends, family and doctors.

---

* The Truth About Cancer (TTAC) and The Quest for the Cures; Bollinger, Ty and Charlene; Convention and Video Series; *The Quest for the Cures*, 2014; et al.,; *A Global Quest*, 2015; Et al.,; *Eastern Medicine; Journey through Asia*, 2018; et al.; The Truth about Vaccines; et al.,; *A Life Saving Mission* (Anaheim, CA, October 11–13, 2019); Truth about Cancer Live (Nashville, TN, October 22–24, 2021), https://thetruthaboutcancer.com/category/videos/.

† Life Extension. *The Science of a Healthier Life*, Journal Articles *The Power of Plant Based Nutrients* (October 2021).

CANCER PREVENTION

Here are some tips you may or may not have implemented.

1. Avoid known carcinogens, chemicals, and toxins. Get a heavy metals test and learn how to detoxify.
2. Drink clean water. No chlorine, which kills natural intestinal bacteria and downregulates your immune system. Mineralize your water.
3. Eat organic raw fruits and vegetables only. This prevents organ exhaustion and gastrointestinal enzyme depletion.
4. Supplement with digestive enzymes. These help the healing process after surgery.* Supplement friendly bacteria with probiotics and prebiotics, including *S. boulardii*, a beneficial yeast.
5. Consume little or no sugar and sweets, which weaken the immune system. Also, avoid glutamine.
6. Adopt a regular exercise routine. Learn how to breathe to shift your system away from sympathetic overdrive using Wim Hof and Buteyko breathing.†
7. Remove from the bowel using a cleansing program.
8. Laugh, love, and think positively. This increases natural killer cells (NKCs).
9. Use PQQ and serotonin, abundantly. PQQ targets multiple cell-signaling pathways that are directly involved in the upregulation of cellular energy metabolism and causes mitochondrial biogenesis. Serotonin at 120 mg inhibits metallo-proteinase-9 and is antiviral, antibacterial, and anticancer.
10. Follow a program of targeted nutritionals. See the Appendix, and add vitamin B17.
11. 7-Keto DHEA activates natural killer cells (NKCs).
12. Graviola can wipe out twelve types of cancer cells, including breast, prostate, colon, lung, and pancreatic tumors.
13. Take in at least three to five servings of fruits and vegetables daily.
14. When your cellular voltage drops, that is when cancer begins. Dental infected areas have low voltage. When the voltage hits +30 mV then cancer takes over. Normal voltage in the cellular membrane is -20 to-25 millivolts.‡ PHI is elevated in cancer. This is an enzyme that regulates the metastatic spread of cancer. Most cancers are usually flatlined until progesterone drops. So, check your progesterone hormone levels.
15. Keep your insulin levels low! The lower the better.

---

* A4M Advanced Hands-On Intensive Physician Clinical Workshop (Las Vegas, NV, May 13–15, 2005).

† Wim Hof, *The Wim Hof Method: Activate Your Full Human Potential* (Sounds True, June 28, 2022).

‡ Tennant, *Healing Is Voltage.*

Folic Acid and Cancer

Low levels of folic acid have been implicated in the increased risk of several cancers, including colon, lung, and cervical cancer. Women who consume diets low in folic acid are at an increased risk for developing cervical dysplasia and cancer of the cervix, whereas optimal folic acid intake appears to prevent precancerous conditions of the cervix. Gregorios Paspatis, MD, at the Metaxa Cancer Hospital in Piraeus, Greece, reports that low levels of folic acid increase the risk of colon adenomas, a type of colon tumor.[*] Folic acid deficiency causes cellular damage that resembles the initial stages of cancer, whereas optimal folic acid status may prevent the transformation of abnormal cells into cancerous cells.

If you are suspecting cancer, explore these potential alternative explanations:

- Heavy metal toxicity
- Dental infections
- Increased stress
- Low voltage (voltage below + 30 mV) is considered the start of cancer progression
- Parasites[†] (cloves, wormwood, and black walnut are antiparasitic and help to rid you of parasitic bacteria)[‡, §]

Boron and Cancer

New studies have shown that 3 mg of boron daily has demonstrated bone remineralization and anticancer properties, especially lung, prostatic, and HPV or cervical cancer. Boron disrupts the cycle of the human papillomavirus (HPV), a contributing factor to almost 95 percent of all cervical cancers. HPV also occurs in your mouth and is causative for a number of oral conditions. We have boron in our formulation called Pearl Silica Drops®.

A Few More Cancer Facts

You must change the biological terrain to effect a real change in your cancer journey. Bio-oxidative and ozone therapy is the best bang for your buck.

All cancers have fungus before cancer occurs; the fungal infections are usually present for two years prior to cancer development. This is what the PSA

---

* Gregorios Paspatis, MD, "Folate status and adenomatous colonic polyps. A colonoscopically controlled study," https://pubmed.ncbi.nlm.nih.gov/7813348/.

† Dr. Lee Merritt, Parasites, Cancer, and Autoimmune Disease, http://www.shelleybholisticnutrition.com/post/dr-lee-merritt-on-parasites-cancer-autoimmune-disease

‡ Dr. Josh Axe, Ty Bollinger, Jordan Rubin, *Essential Oils, Ancient Medicine,* (Axe Wellness, LLC, 2016).

§ Connie and Alan Higley, *Quick Reference Guide to Using Essential Oils* (Abundant Health, 2016).

marker indicates. That is, the amount of fungus in your prostate gland, and *not* the degree of cancer. Celebrex has been shown to stop prostate cancer.

In periodontal disease, when the voltage drops and oxygen becomes depleted, the cell spirochetes come out of the red blood cells and invade healthy tissues. Most all cancers are flatlined and when progesterone levels drop, cancer appears.*

Melatonin is a premier anticancer nutrient, especially for oral cancer, according to Dr. Frank Shallenberger.† It decreases osteoclastic bone activity, is a potent CNS oxidative scavenger, decreases periodontal bone loss, decreases TNF-alpha, and stops the growth of cancer.

Cancer Supplementation

Natural Cancer Therapies Are Very Effective

Cancer is a multifactorial disease. It is estimated that 90 percent of all cancers are influenced by lifestyle and nutrition, yet science is still looking for that magic bullet that will somehow cure cancer with a prescription drug.

If I were you, I wouldn't wait for their magic bullet, I would start right now with the listing below:

1. Curcumin, also called turmeric, stops precancerous tissue growth. It promotes cellular apoptosis; must be taken with piperine.
2. Preconditioning with ozone gas by insufflation or injection. You need your own machine for this.
3. Vitamin D3. Get your levels up to 80 to 100 ng/dl.
4. IV vitamin C therapy causes oxygenation of cancer cells. Oxygen to the cell wall causes the cell membranes to become more permeable and thus, they explode. This H_2O_2 only affects the cancer cells.
5. Barley grass is a food that assists in cellular membrane oxygenation.
6. 5-Lox inhibitors.
7. An anti-inflammatory diet, follow the list.
8. Follow the "Steps to Alkalinize" list.
9. Active hexose correlated compound (AHCC), an active mushroom extract.
10. Get rid of your dental infections; they are screwing up your voltage.
11. Apigenin slows the progression of breast cancer.
12. Bell peppers contain over thirty carotenoids.
13. Omega-3 fatty acids, seven grams per day.
14. TA-65 MD, for lengthening telomeres, cell rejuvenation through telomerase activation from: soy isoflavones (genistein and diadzein).

---

* Dr. Mark Rosenberg, MD, A4M 24th Annual World Congress on Anti-Aging Medicine, conference notes (Hollywood, FL, May 20–21, 2016).

† Frank Shallenberger, MD, HMD, *The Ozone Miracle*, 2017.

These inhibit angiogenesis and block tyrosine kinase, an enzyme which promotes the growth of tumor cells.

15. Progesterone supplementation, bioidentical or oral-micronized.
16. Alkaline water, Vollara or use H+ water, or Kangen water and a Berkey or a ProOne filter.
17. Follow the 80 percent alkaline diet sheet (see Appendix 2).
18. Elimination of all sugar sources; this shuts off glycolysis, which is the pathway that feeds cancer.
19. Green tea extract, ECGC.
20. Chlorogenic acid, green coffee bean extract.
21. Turkey-tail mushroom extracts; these contain beta-glucans which release antitumor messengers.
22. Sulphoraphane, contained in cruciferous vegetables.
23. Poly-MVA may diminish cancerous tumors.
24. A baked apple in the morning contains quercetin. Eat the skin but make sure it is organic.
25. Iodine, an alkalinizing substance, at least 12.5 mgs per day.
26. Protandim, a blend of five different herbs that increase glutathione, SOD, and catalase.
27. Astaxanthin.
28. Oatmeal (also contain beta glucans).
29. Peaches (the Rich Lady variety) contain polyphenols which kills breast cancer cells.
30. Plums (the Black Splendor variety).
31. Ozone-10 pass, also called auto-hemolytic therapy and now ozone dialysis.

Eat your veggies, they are electron donors and they are alkaline and increase the cellular voltage. Balance all of your hormones with a complete hormone panel. (ZRT test kit)

Metformin is probably the best Big Pharma diabetes drug. It is the #1 prescribed oral hyperglycemic drug for diabetes, and it has been shown to decrease some cancers, especially prostate cancer.

Butyrate is a fiber compound found in beans that inactivates IL-6. IL-6 is found in high levels in cancer cells and in periodontal disease. It is an inflammatory cytokine that is produced in the liver.

BEC, also called Cureaderm,* is an Australian skin cream for melanoma treatment. Also use black topical salve† for smaller skin cancer lesions.

---

* BEC5, Curacerm, http://www.bec5curaderm.com/.

† Alpha Omega Labs, http://www.herbhealers.com/.

NATURAL CANCER THERAPIES

Dosing to be determined by your health practitioner. It's all about changing the biological terrain.

- CBD oil, full spectrum and micellized for better cellular absorption.
- Chia seed oil and omega-3, -7, -9 oil, and celery sticks.
- Far-infrared sauna therapy.
- PEMF Mat. I use the i-MRS Mat.
- Medi Air Purifier Ozone Ionizer.
- Ozone generator (in home).
- Ozone auto-hemolytic therapy. Contact AAOT for doctors in your area.
- Black seed oil: one teaspoon per day.
- IV vitamin C injections.
- Vitamin C liposomal, or ascorbyl palmitate-C.
- Liposomal glutathione.
- Green tea extract, EGCG.
- Iodine complex 25 mg per day (Iodoral).
- Selenium, Triple from Life Extension.
- Enhanced DIM, Douglass Labs.
- Essential oils, especially frankincense, which is also called Boswellia.
- MCT oil (coconut oil), one tablespoon per day.
- Argentyn-23®, daily.
- Ozone gas and ozone water.
- Hyper-Oxy Ozone Sticks.
- Melatonin Max, 120 mg per day from SHS, Scientific Health Solutions.
- Poly-MVA, will diminish tumor size.
- Modified citrus pectin.
- Graviola.
- Turmeric, curcumin.
- Alkaline greens.
- Trans-resveratrol (I take this with omega-3 EFAs).
- AHCC.
- Black topical salve.
- PQQ, 20 to 40 mg a day.
- Strict ketogenic diet.*
- Absolutely no sugar or glutamine.
- Vitamin D3 21,000 IUs per day (my dosing regimen).

---

* Toni Bark, MD, The Truth About Cancer, TTAC, *A Life Saving Mission* (Anaheim, CA, October 11–13, 2019).

A WORD ABOUT RDA DOSING OF SUPPLEMENTS

When it comes to oral supplementation of vitamins and minerals, there are some principles you need to be aware of concerning the recommended daily allowance numbers. First off, you need to know that these government-recommended daily allowances are set at extremely low levels. For example, in the case of vitamin C, the RDA is set at a level just high enough to prevent scurvy in rats. Secondly, when you consume, say, 1000 mgs of vitamin C by mouth, at least half of it becomes conjugated by the liver as it passes through the digestive system, so the total amount of the vitamin C left that is available for use is 500 mgs, as you lose 50 percent in the digestive process.

The following appendixes consist of the majority of my antiaging suggestions. This will get you started on the right track. Exercise, proper sleep, and positive thinking, probiotics and *S. boulardii*, of course, would be other suggestions.

—God Bless and Good Health~
Dr. Thom

APPENDIX 1

Anti-Inflammatory Foods

Take this list with you when you go shopping

Protein Sources
Raw milk and dairy
GMO-free eggs
Wild cod, some acidity
Wild salmon, some acidity
Wild-game meats

Carbohydrates
Green beans
Kidney beans
Oatmeal (old-fashioned organic)
Pumpkin
Squash
Sweet potato
Wild rice, very alkaline
Yams

Healthy Fats
Avocado
Chia seeds
Cold-water fish
Flaxseed oil
Nuts
Olives and olive oil
Pumpkin seeds
Coconut oil

Vegetarian Protein
Seitan
Soy foods, *fermented only*
Tofu, *fermented only*
Tempeh
Texturized vegetable protein
Veggie burgers (homemade only)

Fruits
Apples
Apricots
Bananas
Blueberries
Cantaloupe
Dates
Figs
Grapes
Grapefruit
Kiwi
Lemons and limes
Oranges (including mandarin and tangerines)
Peaches
Pears
Pineapple
Prunes
Raisins

Vegetables
Asparagus
Artichoke
Broccoli
Brussel Sprouts
Carrots
Cauliflower
Celery
Cucumber
Garlic
Green beans
Peppers
Leafy greens
Lettuce
Onions
Peas
Pea pods
Peppers
Spinach
Zucchini

FOODS TO AVOID
High-fructose corn syrup
All trans-fats
(especially canola oil)
All seed oils
Fried foods
Mayonnaise
Low-fat dairy products
All wheat products
All GMO products
All boxed foods
All microwaveable foods
All low-fat products
Margarine
Skim milk

Low glycemic index/load (GI/GL) foods:

Proteins:
- Eggs
- Fish (especially cold-water fish like salmon)
- Poultry (chicken, turkey)
- Lean cuts of meat
- Tofu
- Tempeh

Legumes:
- Lentils
- Chickpeas
- Black beans
- Kidney beans

Non-Starchy Vegetables:
- Broccoli
- Spinach
- Kale
- Cauliflower
- Green beans
- Bell peppers
- Leafy greens (lettuce, arugula, Swiss chard)
- Cucumber
- Zucchini

Whole Grains:
- Quinoa
- Barley
- Buckwheat
- Oats (steel-cut or rolled)

Nuts and Seeds:
- Almonds
- Walnuts
- Chia seeds
- Flaxseeds
- Pumpkin seeds

Fruits:

- Berries (strawberries, blueberries, raspberries)
- Cherries
- Grapefruit
- Apples
- Pears

Healthy Fats:

- Avocado
- Olive oil
- Coconut oil
- Nuts and seeds (in moderation)

Controlling insulin also depends on the PR to CHO ratio.

High-dose omega-3 oil decreases silent inflammation and increases wellness in:

1. Heart disease
2. Cancer
3. Bipolar depression (10 g a day, begets a 500 percent greater reversal)
4. ADD, ADHD
5. Multiple Sclerosis
6. Alzheimer's
7. Chronic pain
8. Skin disorders
9. Autoimmune disease
10. Brain dysfunction
11. Pain and arthritis control.

How Much Omega-3 Oil Do You Need?

- Maintenance dosing = 3 grams per day (1 tbsp of cod liver oil)
- Improving heart function = 5 grams per day
- For chronic pain = 7.5 grams per day
- For Neurological disease = 10 grams per day or more

Note: The more you control insulin, the less omega-3s you need; the less you control insulin, the more omega-3s you need.

APPENDIX 2

Alkaline Foods

Purchase 80 percent of your groceries from this list.

Almonds
Avocado
Bananas
Black olives
Brazil Nuts
Butter (Kerry Gold brand)
Cabbage
Chestnuts
Cold pressed oils, no vegetable oils
Cucumbers
Dates
Green Tea
Green and yellow beans
Mangos
Potatoes (the small purple ones)
Pears
Raisins
Salad greens
Sprouts (all)
Sweet apricots
Sweet pepper
Sweet potatoes
D-Ribose
Xylitol (limited use)
Zucchini

Very Alkaline

Artichokes
Beet greens
Broccoli
Brussel sprouts
Carrots
Celery stalks
Chicory
Dandelion
Escarole
Fennel
Green cabbage
Green beans
Lettuce
Mache
Red beets
Red cabbage
Raw milk
Salad greens
Spinach

APPENDIX 3

Mercury Toxicity Sensitivity Questionnaire

Sore gums (gingivitis)	Yes	No
Mental symptoms such as confusion, forgetfulness	Yes	No
Severe depression	Yes	No
Ringing in the ears (tinnitus)	Yes	No
TMJ (Temporal Mandibular Joint) problems	Yes	No
Unusual shakiness (tremors) of hands or arms	Yes	No
Brown spots or aging spots	Yes	No
Colds, flu, infectious diseases	Yes	No
Food allergies or intolerances	Yes	No
Have you been to many doctors regarding your health	Yes	No
Numbness, burning in mouth and gums	Yes	No
Numbness or unexplained tingling in arms and legs	Yes	No
Difficulty in walking (ataxia)	Yes	No
Four or more silver or amalgam fillings	Yes	No
A metallic taste in your mouth	Yes	No
Worked as a painter, chemical manufacturing, pesticide (fungicides w/methyl mercury), etc.	Yes	No
Worked as a dentist, hygienist, or dental assistant	Yes	No
Candida Related Complex (CRC) or yeast infections	Yes	No
Bad breath (halitosis) or white tongue (thrush)	Yes	No
Low basal body temperature (below 97.4 degrees F)	Yes	No
Constipation	Yes	No
Heart irregularities or rapid pulse (tachycardia)	Yes	No
Arthritis	Yes	No
Mucus in stools	Yes	No
Chest pains	Yes	No
Poor sleep or insomnia	Yes	No
Frequent kidney infections or kidney problems	Yes	No
Extreme Fatigue	Yes	No

Irritability or dramatic changes in behavior	Yes	No
Using antidepressants or antacids?	Yes	No
Do you have trigeminal neuralgia or other neuralgias?	Yes	No

Scoring Your Test

If you answered yes to three or more questions, you may have hidden toxic metal poisoning.

A toxic metal screening is recommended using the porphyrins test by Metametrix or Doctors Data, and/or the Mercury Tri-Test by Quicksilver Scientific.

APPENDIX 4

TMJ Self-Assessment Questionnaire

1.	Do you have frequent headaches?	Yes	No
2.	Do you hear popping, clicking or cracking sounds when you chew?	Yes	No
3.	Do you hear a grating sound (like crumpling of newspaper) when you chew?	Yes	No
4.	Do you have stuffiness, pressure or blockage in your ears?	Yes	No
5.	Do you hear a ringing or buzzing sound in either or both of your ears?	Yes	No
6.	Do you experience dizziness frequently?	Yes	No
7.	Do your jaws feel like they "catch"?	Yes	No
8.	Do your jaws feel tight, difficult to open?	Yes	No
9.	Does it appear that you can't open your mouth as wide as you used to?	Yes	No
10.	Does your tongue go between your teeth or do you bite on your tongue to keep your teeth apart?	Yes	No
11.	Do your teeth ache?	Yes	No
12.	Are your teeth sensitive, especially to cold temperatures?	Yes	No
13.	Do you wake with sore facial muscles?	Yes	No
14.	Do you clench or grind your teeth during movements of frustration or concentration?	Yes	No
15.	Do you grind your teeth at night?	Yes	No
16.	Do your ears hurt?	Yes	No
17.	Does it hurt to move your jaw sideways?	Yes	No

18. Does your neck, back of your head, or shoulder hurt?	Yes	No
19. Have you been hit in the jaw?	Yes	No
20. Have you been put to sleep for surgery?	Yes	No
21. Have you had a whiplash injury?	Yes	No
22. Have you seen a neurologist, psychologist or psychiatrist for unexplained head or neck pain?	Yes	No
23. Do your jaws ache after eating?	Yes	No
24. Are you under a lot of stress?	Yes	No
25. Have you been told that you might have TMJ?	Yes	No

Scoring Your Test

If you answered yes to five or more questions, you may have a TMJ problem. See a TMJ specialist to discuss whether treatment is called for.

APPENDIX 5

CR or Caloric Reduction

This is the only method scientifically-proven to increase your lifespan. Eating less is one sure way to increase your health and live a longer life. Besides, with the cost of food skyrocketing, you'll save money.

Do you want to spend more time with your kids or grandchildren?
Then do these things:

Eat less food, it means fewer digestive enzymes are required. This has a sparing effect on your metabolic enzymes and helps them to last longer. It also reduces free radical oxidative stress.

There is less lipid peroxidation, thus, less inflammation. So, your cellular membrane integrity improves. This keeps you healthy.

Fasting increases melatonin levels, increases longevity and lowers BMI, resulting in less outpouring of super oxides, which are highly inflammatory. Centenarians have lower lipid peroxide levels. CR: feed animals 1-X per day and they'll live longer with less disease.

CR reduces random aging by decreasing:

1. Free radical oxidative stress
2. Advanced glycosylated end product formation *(AGEs)*
3. Fat accumulation
4. Loss of bone mass
5. Insulin levels
6. Inflammation
7. Heart disease
8. Blood lipid levels (esp., triglycerides)
9. Auto immune disease thereby boosting immunity
10. Blood glucose levels
11. Cancer
12. Diabetes

And by increasing:

13. Enzyme function
14. Immune system function
15. Kidney function
16. Female fertility

APPENDIX 6

The Meridian Tooth Chart

The Meridian Tooth Chart aligns with acupuncture meridians, which are pathways of energy connecting various body parts, glands, and tissues. Each tooth corresponds to a specific meridian, facilitating the flow of energy. Dentists who utilize this chart can often gauge patients' overall health by examining their oral health. If a specific system or organ shows weakness, the condition of the corresponding tooth may potentially worsen the issue.

You can download a PDF of the Tooth Meridian/Dental Organ Relationship Chart from Dr. Yuriy May at Natural Dentistry https://naturaldentistrycenter.com/natural-dentistry/meridian-tooth-chart/.

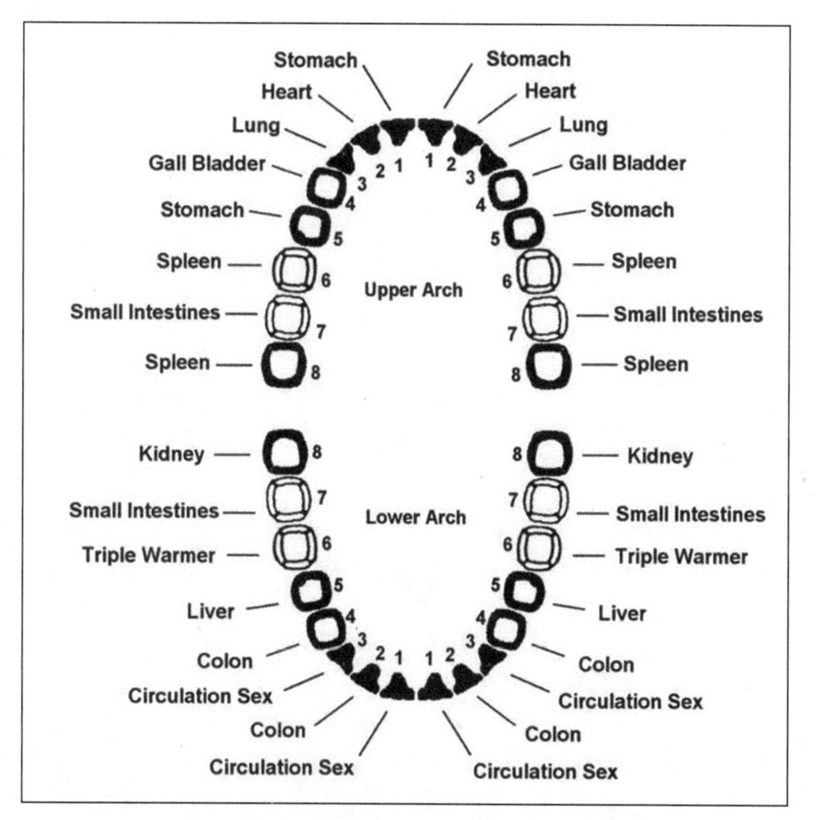

APPENDIX 7

PROBIOTIC and PREBIOTIC INSTRUCTIONS

What do I look for in a probiotic formulation? How much should I take and in what form do I take it? Should it be refrigerated, in liquid form, powdered, etc.? These are all important questions and deserve some consideration.*

LOOK FOR THESE THINGS:

- A reputable, physician grade source. The quality of the probiotics is paramount.
- If you travel, especially overseas, you need to take digestive enzymes and probiotics.
- "If you have a colon, take probiotics." —Brenda Watson CNC
- How many billions of CFU's are left at the time of expiration? There should be 15 to 20 billion units, per strain. This stands for Colony Forming Units.
- The Culture count is the total amount of CFU's in one serving.
- The number of strains in the formulation. There are thousands of bacterial strains. Different strains work in different areas of the body. You need at least 7 strains. More is better.
- At a bare minimum, you need lactobacillus and bifido-bacterium strains.
- At the time of release, they must get through the stomach and be delivered to either the small or large intestines.
- The more strains of bacteria, the better. Some brands have 1 to 2 strains, some have up to 16. Strains and cultures are sometimes used interchangeably. The higher the culture count per strain, the better.

* Source: Brenda Watson, CNC, on Ted Talks.

APPENDIX 8

Dirty Dozen and the Clean 15

The Shopper's Guide includes the Dirty Dozen™ and the Clean Fifteen™—EWG's lists of the most and least pesticide-contaminated conventional fresh fruits and vegetables, respectively, based on results from the latest tests by the Department of Agriculture and the Food and Drug Administration.

Dirty Dozen™

Of the 46 items included in our analysis, these 12 fruits and vegetables were most contaminated with pesticide.

1. Strawberries
2. Spinach
3. Kale, collard, and mustard greens
4. Grapes
5. Peaches
6. Pears
7. Nectarines
8. Apples
9. Bell and hot peppers
10. Cherries
11. Blueberries
12. Green beans

Clean Fifteen™

These 15 items had the lowest amounts of pesticide residues, according to EWG's analysis of the most recent USDA data.

1. Carrots
2. Sweet potatoes
3. Mangoes
4. Mushrooms
5. Watermelon

6. Cabbage
7. Kiwi
8. Honeydew melon
9. Asparagus
10. Sweet peas (frozen)
11. Papaya*
12. Onions
13. Pineapple
14. Sweet corn*
15. Avocados

* A small amount of sweet corn, papaya and summer squash sold in the United States is produced from genetically modified seeds. Buy organic varieties of these crops if you want to avoid genetically modified produce.*

* Environmental Working Group (EWG), https://http://www.food-safety.com/articles/9329-ewg-publishes-2024-dirty-dozen-list-of-produce-most- contaminated-with-pesticides.

APPENDIX 9

A Final Word

So, What Must I Take?

This is my very abridged version of what you must take as an antiaging regimen to stay reasonably healthy.

Here is what I recommend. Most supplements are available on my website at the DSS Store.[*]

1. Omega-3, -7, and -9, EFAs (healthy fats) (I use Dr. Sinatra's[†])
2. Nattokinase and Serratopeptidase
3. Boost your nitric oxide levels with Cardio Miracle®, a heart-healthy nitric oxide booster[‡, §]
4. Corvalen D-ribose, as directed
5. Iodine (Iodoral®) at least 12.5 mg per day
6. Selenium, three types in one blend by Life Extension
7. GTA Forte, from Biotics, this is pure T-3[¶]
8. Perfect Aminos[**] (eight essential amino acids)
9. Balance your hormones and neurotransmitters[††]
10. Increase your parasympathetic nervous system (PSNS) by learning how to breathe through your nose, Wim Hof[‡‡] or Buteyko breathing method.[§§]

---

* http://www.drlokensgard.com/supplements.

† http://www.healthydirections.com/product-categories/dr-sinatra.

‡ Et al., http://www.CardioMiracle.com.

§ Scott Laird, ND, and Jodi Laird; Laird Wellness; https://rumble.com/v31sisg-nitric-oxide-the-miracle-molecule.html.

¶ https://shop.bioticsresearch.com/collections/all-products-a-z.

** https://bodyhealth.com/.

†† Scott Laird, ND, Laird Wellness, http://www.lairdwellness.com.

‡‡ Wim Hof, *The Wim Hof Method: Activate Your Full Human Potential* (Sounds True, June 28, 2022).

§§ Ralph Skuban, PhD, *The Buteyko Method: How to Improve Your Breathing for Better Health and Performance in All Areas of Life*, based on 1960s research by Ukrainian physician Dr.

11. Take multi-probiotics and digestive enzymes daily (Laird Wellness or Ancient Nutrition)
12. NAC, 1200 mg per day
13. DIM Enhanced, by Douglas Labs
14. Decrease NF-kappa Beta
15. Take a serving of greens every day
16. Increase your nitric oxide levels and protect your heart[*]
17. Take L-Citrulline, L-Ornithine & L-Arginine to help increase nitric oxide levels
18. PQQ and Mitochondrial Energy Optimizer
19. Take NAD+, and Pearl Silica Drops® daily
20. Take collagen bone broth; I use Ancient Nutrition[†]
21. Follow the ketogenic diet, by Dr. Toni Bark, MD
22. CR; caloric reduction approach (eat less). This increases mitochondrial biogenesis.
23. Drink Pure H2O with Concentrace® Trace Mineral Drops (twenty-one drops)[‡]
24. Also add six to ten drops of Pearl Silica Drops®[§]
25. Trans-resveratrol, as this increases Sirt-1 and Sirt-2
26. Green tea extract, EGCG
27. Magnesium-L-threonate, 1200 mg a day
28. Vitamin D3, 14000 IUs per day
29. Liposomal glutathione
30. Liposomal vitamin C, 3000 mg daily
31. A full-spectrum B-complex vitamin formulation
32. IntraMax® all-in-one Liquid Vitamins (Drucker Labs) (IntraKid® for children)
33. Melatonin (max 180 mg per day), it is anticancer, from SHS
34. NT-Factor Energy Lipids ARG (glyco-phospholipids), for your cell membranes.

Konstantin Buteyko, 1923–2003 (Skuban Academy; 1st edition (February 14, 2024).

[*] http://www.CardioMiracle.com.

[†] https://ancientnutrition.com.

[‡] Concentrace® Trace Mineral Drops; http://http://www.traceminerals.com.

[§] https://pearloralhealth.com/.

APPENDIX 10

The Life Rejuvenation Programs

There are two Life Rejuvenation programs developed by the author. The first is the naturopathic medical program which consists of twenty-one Self-Help Modules. The second is the Fourteen-Modular Oral Biological Dentistry Program for the dentistry professionals and patients alike. The modules include natural scientific medical approaches for your health.

THE LIFE REJUVENATION LIFE ENHANCEMENT PROGRAMS

1) The Age Rejuvenation Life Enhancement Program

A Complete and Comprehensive Twenty-One-Modular Self-Help Program for Obtaining and Maintaining Optimal Health and Wellness for Everyone. The Contents of the Age-Rejuvenation Naturopathic Medical Program includes:

The Core Seven-Step Program:

1. Silent Inflammation and NFK beta Control
2. Digestive System and the Organs of Elimination
3. Brain, Bioenergy and Neurotransmitter Systems
4. Cardiovascular System and Mitochondrial Energy Support
5. Glandular-Hormonal Endocrine Optimization
6. Muscular and Skeletal Support Systems
7. Immunity, DNA-Repair, and Chromosomal Protection

The Fourteen Related Sub-Modules:

8. How Come I Can't Sleep, Snoring and OSA (Obstructive Sleep Apnea)
9. Biological Dentistry and Oral Health
10. Your Gut Repair Kit
11. Whole-Body Detoxification
12. The Metabolic Syndrome and Blood Sugar Control
13. Your Waist-Disposal Program (Total Weight Control)
14. The New Antiaging Report Card
15. Dietary Endocrinology and Nutri-Genomics

16. Thyroid and Adrenal Function
17. Read Your Own Labs
18. Your Vitamin, Mineral, and Antioxidant Manual
19. Diseases and Their Natural Treatments
20. The Sensory Organs, Skin, Optic, Audiology
21. Natural Cancer Therapies

2) The Oral Biological Dentistry Enhancement Program Contents:
The contents of this program consists of fourteen modules of self-help instruction and was designed for medical and dentistry healthcare professionals, as well as engaged laypersons on their journey to learn more about biological and holistic dentistry. I wish you all well in your journey.

The Core Seven-Step Program includes:

1. Biological Dentistry and Silent Inflammation, NF-K Beta
2. Facial Rejuvenation and Cosmetic Dentistry
3. Snoring, Insomnia, and Osa Splints
4. Orthopedic Orthodontics and Facial Growth
5. TMD, Headaches, and Appliances
6. Dentures, Implants, and Restorative Dentistry
7. Natural Nutrient Regimens for Dentistry

The seven related modules include:

8. Doctor's Bio-Dentistry Business Model
9. Heavy Metal and Whole-Body Detoxification Program
10. Periodontal Disease and Cardiovascular Disease
11. Read Your Own Labs and Bio-Inflammatory Markers
12. Patient's Guide to Better Oral Health
13. All Biological Dentistry Consent Forms
14. The Remineralization Protocol for Teeth and Bone

Acknowledgments

To my incredible patients, thank you for trusting me and allowing me into your lives, getting to know you, your families, your kiddos, and sometimes working through difficult clinical situations.

It has been my honor to have worked with you and to have served and assisted you with your healthcare needs!

Thanks also for teaching me many valuable lifetime lessons. I've learned so much from all of you.

To my friends, Greg, Julie, and Nancy Webster, who assisted greatly in the writing and the motivation for bringing this book to fruition, which would not have been written without them! This book is dedicated to Greg, who has gone to be with the Lord.

To my staff, thank you for your overwhelming support in caring for our patients. You have supported me throughout this whole endeavor, and I can't thank you enough. You've even suffered through all of my jokes! You gave me support when I needed it the most, and for that I am truly grateful and honored.

This book is also dedicated to my beautiful wife, Jan, who is a blessing and who gives me continued inspiration and a reason to "get it right." Thanks for putting up with me during this and my many other projects throughout our journey. You continue to be my inspiration!

And to the memories of James and Sally Lokensgard (Gardner) and Clayton Gardner, the three people who influenced my life in a most positive way. May they rest in peace until we are all reunited in heaven! I miss you!

And lastly, but most importantly, is the overall help, guidance, and Divine intervention from our heavenly Creator also known as "the Great Physician," and Yeshua, His son, whom it has been my honor to serve.

Thank you and blessings to you all!
Dr. Thom

Index

A

Abraham, Guy, 96
active hexose correlated compound (AHCC), 180, 182
adenosine triphosphate (ATP), 11, 19, 53, 57, 99, 177
age rejuvenation, 7
AHCC. *See* active hexose correlated compound (AHCC)
air pollution, 106
airway space, 24
alkalinity, 12, 26, 30, 31, 32, 33, 46, 53, 98–101, 111, 180, 189
alpha amylase, 36
aluminum, 30, 101, 106, 160
Alzheimer's disease, 24, 29–30
Amiel, Henri Frederick, 6
antacids, 16
antiaging medicine, 49–62
antibiotics, 41, 137, 163
antibodies, 40, 72, 95, 130, 139, 176
anticoagulant therapy, 40
antioxidants, 9, 28–29, 37, 38, 66, 98, 153
antiphospholipid syndrome, 40
apigenin, 180
Argentyn 23, 30, 32, 33, 73, 141, 145, 151, 163, 182
ATP. *See* adenosine triphosphate (ATP)
autism, 22, 147, 149, 152, 153, 155, 159–160
Auto-Hemolytic Therapy, 24

B

babies, 71–73
Baltimore, David, 80
BDNF. *See* brain-derived neurogenic factor (BDNF)
betaine hydrochloride, 13
bifidus factor, 95
BIHRT. *See* bioidentical hormone replacement therapy (BIHRT)
biofilm, 45–47
bioidentical hormone replacement therapy (BIHRT), 50
bio-impedance analysis (BIA), 13
biological stressors, 8–9
biological systems, 8
blood vessels, chelation and, 154
B-lymphocytes, 95
bone remineralization, 164–167
boron, 165, 179
brain-derived neurogenic factor (BDNF), 54
breastfeeding, 72–73, 167–168
breath, bad, 32–34
bruxism, 78

C

calcium, 115, 165
caloric restriction (CR), 13, 42, 43, 87
cancer, 17, 33, 44, 65, 98, 109, 127, 175–183
cancer supplementation, 180–182
candida, 7, 137–146
carbohydrates, 17. *See also* sugar
cellular healing protocol, 11–14
cellular metabolic medicine (CMM), 14
chelation therapy, 68, 154–156
chewing, 24
cholesterol, 12, 16, 96, 154, 164
chromosomal support, 164
CLA. *See* conjugated linoleic acid (CLA)
CMM. *See* cellular metabolic medicine (CMM)
coenzyme Q10, 12, 31
colon, in elimination, 156–157
conjugated linoleic acid (CLA), 95

constipation, 133–135
CR. *See* caloric restriction (CR)
craniofacial orthopedics, 55–58
craniosacral therapy, 61–62
Crean, St. John, 29
curcumin, 180
cytokines, 11, 43, 69, 83, 139, 181. *See also* inflammation

D

decay, dental, 20–27, 45–47
dentinal fluid transport system (DFTS), 24–27, 45–47
dentinal lymph fluid (DLF), 26, 27
deodorant, 106–107
detoxification, 16, 22, 68, 149–159
DFTS. *See* dentinal fluid transport system (DFTS)
diet. *See also* caloric restriction (CR)
  alkaline, 189
  anti-inflammatory, 86–87, 185–187
  biblical, 89–91
  fats in, 85–86
  inflammation and, 80
  ketogenic, 71
  myths of, 16, 17
  pain-free, 77
  standard American, 17, 80, 86, 147, 163
  sugar in, 27
DLF. *See* dentinal lymph fluid (DLF)
d-ribose, 12

E

ECM. *See* extracellular matrix (ECM)
endocannabinoid system, 100
ENOS, 66
enzymes, digestive, 13
extracellular matrix (ECM), 9
extractions, 40

F

Fallon, Sally, 94
fat cells, 42, 130. *See also* obesity
fats, 17
  essential, 12
  low-fat foods, 94, 96, 104, 125–127, 128, 129–131
  omega, 85–86, 131, 180
fibronectin, 95
fillings, 22, 72, 152–153. *See also* mercury
FJOs. *See* functional jaw orthopedics (FJOs)
Flechas, Jorge, 96
flossing, 32
fluoride, 16, 72, 93, 108–111
folic acid, 179
FOS. *See* fructooligosaccharides (FOS)
free radicals, 37, 50
fructooligosaccharides (FOS), 13
fulvic acid, 12
functional dentistry
  defined, 4–5
  integrative medicine *vs.*, 3–18
functional jaw orthopedics (FJOs), 58–59
fungus, cancer and, 179–180

G

galvanic currents, 24
gastric reflux, 32
genetically modified organisms (GMOs), 111–113
GI. *See* glycemic index (GI)
gingivitis, 27–29, 30–32
GL. *See* glycemic load (GL)
glutamate, 127
glutathione, 22, 72, 77, 151, 153
glycemic index (GI), 87–89
glycemic load (GL), 87–89
glycosphingolipids, 95
GMOs. *See* genetically modified organisms (GMOs)
Gordon, Gay, 68
Greenberg, Robert, 9
gum, 31, 34

H

health, roots of, 6–8
heart, 20
heartburn, 16, 81
heart rate variability (HRV), 54, 78
homeopathic injections, 40
hormonal levels, 50, 95
HRV. *See* heart rate variability (HRV)
hs-CRP, 23

Huber, Don, 111
humic acid, 12
hyaline, 36
hyberbaric therapy, 40
hydration, 12, 13
hypo-fibrinolysis, 40
hypothyroidism, 108

I

IAOMT Protocol, 4
implants, dental, 24
infants, 71–73
infections, 23, 66
  acidification and, 98
  cancer and, 176, 179–180
  candida, 137, 138, 139, 140
  cavitations and, 39
  charge and, 46, 66
  middle ear, 31
  oil pulling and, 69
  oxygenation and, 44–45
  root canal and, 40, 43
  voltage and, 44–45
  xylitol and, 114
inflammation, 4, 20–21, 43, 69, 79–91, 185–187. *See also* cytokines
insulin, 104, 112, 127, 130
integrative medicine, 3–18
iodine, 12, 16, 30, 96–98, 110–111, 165, 182
iron, 94, 165

K

Krauthammer, Charles, 79
Krebs cycle, 11, 57

L

lactoferrin, 94
lactoperoxidase, 94
Laird, Scott, 84, 111
LaLanne, Jack, 4
Langevin, Helen, 168
Langley-Evans, Simon, 29
liver, 11, 12, 23, 157
lymphatic system, 36, 37–38, 151, 157, 158. *See also* dentinal fluid transport system (DFTS)
lymph node, 42
lysozymes, 95

M

macrophages, 95
magnesium, 12, 17, 68, 73, 78, 103, 104, 120, 134, 135, 149
McNamara, James, 60
MCTs. *See* medium chain triglycerides (MCTs)
medium chain triglycerides (MCTs), 95
melatonin, 180
mercury, 17, 21, 22, 23, 24, 30, 72, 110, 147–149, 160, 165. *See also* metals, heavy
meridians, dental, 44, 168–169
metals, heavy, 4, 67, 68, 145, 147–159. *See also* mercury
metformin, 181
microbiome, 9
milk, raw, 93–96
mineralization, 46–47, 164–167
minerals, in salt, 103
mitochondria, 8, 9, 11, 12, 13, 14, 55, 83, 99, 140, 160, 174, 178
molars, 40, 44
mucin, 36, 95
myths, 16–18

N

neutrophils, 95
NF-kB. *See* nuclear factor kappa Beta (NF-kB)
NICO lesions, 38
NT factor, 12
nuclear factor kappa Beta (NF-kB), 20, 54, 79
nutritional deficiencies, 45–47

O

obesity, 53, 85, 86, 125–131. *See also* weight control
obstructive sleep apnea (OSA), 5, 24, 55, 56, 77, 84, 117–119
odontoblastic tubules, 43
oil pulling, 30, 69–70
oligosaccharides, 95

omega fats, 85–86, 131, 180
organic, 17
orthodontics, 17
orthopedics, 55–58
OSA. *See* obstructive sleep apnea (OSA)
osteo-cavitations, 24, 38–41
osteonecrosis, 38–39
oxidative stress, 10, 36, 38, 49, 54
oxygen consumption, 19–20
OxyMist, 32, 34, 72, 145, 176
ozone oil, 31, 67
ozone therapy, 41, 46, 65–67, 175, 180, 182

P

pancreas, 36, 38, 127
parotid gland, 27
parotid hormone, 27
Paspatis, Gregorios, 179
PCBs. *See* polychlorinated biphenyls (PCBs)
periodontal disease, 24, 27–29, 30–32
personal care products, 106–107
phosphoric acid, 127
phosphorus, 165
pituitary gland, 26
polychlorinated biphenyls (PCBs), 107–108
polysaccharides, 94
Porphyromonas gingivalis (Pg), 29
potassium, 103, 104
Price, Weston, 46, 94
probiotics, 13, 31, 33, 144, 163
propylene glycol, 106
protein rich plasma (PRP), 40
PRP. *See* protein rich plasma (PRP)
pulpitis, 44

R

reactive oxygen species (ROS), 66
riboflavin, 110
R-lipoic acid, 110
root canals, 23, 24, 40, 43–45
ROS. *See* reactive oxygen species (ROS)

S

salt, 12, 16, 30–31, 101–104, 111
SCT. *See* serum compatibility testing (SCT)
Sears, Al, 176
Sears, Barry, 79
selenium, 12, 54, 100, 103, 141, 165, 166, 177
serum compatibility testing (SCT), 73–74
Servan-Schreiber, David, 175
Shallenberger, Frank, 180
silica, 12, 31
silver hydrosol, 30
Singer, Leon, 110
sleep, 5, 24, 55, 56, 77, 84, 117–121
Soda Doping, 100–101
Sonicare, 31
sphenoid bone, 61–62
sucrose, 27
sugar, 27, 32, 33, 111–115, 126–127, 128–129
sunlight, 13
surgical trauma, 39
Sutherland, William G., 61

T

teething, 72
teeth straightening, 171–173
temporomandibular disorder (TMD), 5, 24, 58, 62, 75–78
Tennant, Jerry, 11, 13
testosterone, 12
tests, 10
thimerosal, 160
thrombophilia, 40
T-lymphocytes, 95
TMD. *See* temporomandibular disorder (TMD)
tongue scraper, 31
toothpaste, 27, 46, 73, 81, 106, 108, 109, 151, 167
toxins, 105–111
truly healthful living (THL), 105
Truss, Orian, 138
Tylenol, 22

U

urinary filtrate, 41–43

V

vaccines, 17, 30, 154, 160

veganism, 16
vegetables, 12
vitamin B2, 110
vitamin B12-binding protein, 95
vitamin C, 180, 183
vitamin D3, 180, 182
voltage, 11–12, 13–14, 42, 44–45, 180

W

water, 12, 17, 31, 53, 110, 115–116, 135, 165
water pollution, 106
WBCs. *See* white blood cells (WBCs)
weight control, 159
White, Reggie, 117
white blood cells (WBCs), 95, 176
Woeller, Kurt, 159
Woodside, Donald, 60

X

xylitol, 113, 114, 115
xylitol gum, 31, 34

Y

yeast. *See* candida

Z

zeolites, 67–69
zinc, 19, 22, 67, 103, 139, 141, 165, 166